Practical Approach to Paediatric Gastroenterology, Hepatology and Nutrition

Practical Approach to Paediatric Gastroenterology, Hepatology and Nutrition

Deirdre Kelly, MD, FRCP, FRCPI, FRCPH

The Liver Unit
Birmingham Children's Hospital;
Professor of Paediatric Hepatology
University of Birmingham
Birmingham, UK

Ronald Bremner, DM, FRCPCH

Consultant Paediatric Gastroenterologist
Department of Gastroenterology and Nutrition
Birmingham Children's Hospital
Birmingham, UK

Jane Hartley, MBChB, MRCPCH, MMedSc, PhD

Consultant in Paediatric Hepatology and Small Bowel Transplantation
The Liver Unit
Birmingham Children's Hospital
Birmingham, UK

Diana Flynn, MBBCh, MRCPCH, BSc, PhD

Consultant Paediatric Gastroenterologist
Department of Gastroenterology
Royal Hospital for Sick Children
Glasgow, UK

WILEY Blackwell

Registered office: John Wiley & Sons, Ltd, The Atrium, Southern Gate, Chichester, West
        Sussex, PO19 8SQ, UK
Editorial offices: 9600 Garsington Road, Oxford, OX4 2DQ, UK
        The Atrium, Southern Gate, Chichester, West Sussex, PO19 8SQ, UK
        111 River Street, Hoboken, NJ 07030-5774, USA

For details of our global editorial offices, for customer services and for information about
how to apply for permission to reuse the copyright material in this book please see our
website at www.wiley.com/wiley-blackwell

Library of Congress Cataloging-in-Publication Data

Bremner, Ronald, author.
  Practical approach to paediatric gastroenterology, hepatology, and nutrition /
Ronald Bremner, Jane Hartley, Diana Flynn ; editor, Deirdre Kelly.
      p. ; cm.
  Includes bibliographical references and index.
  ISBN 978-0-470-67314-0 (pbk. : alk. paper) – ISBN 978-1-118-77866-1 (epdf) –
ISBN 978-1-118-77882-1 (epub) – ISBN 978-1-118-77883-8 (emobi)
  I. Hartley, Jane, author.   II. Flynn, Diana, author.   III. Kelly, Deirdre A., editor.   IV. Title.
  [DNLM: 1. Gastrointestinal Diseases–Handbooks.   2. Child Nutrition Disorders–
Handbooks.   3. Child.   4. Infant Nutrition Disorders–Handbooks.   5. Infant.   6. Liver
Diseases–Handbooks. WS 39]
  RJ446
  618.92'33–dc23

                                        2013024997

A catalogue record for this book is available from the British Library.

Wiley also publishes its books in a variety of electronic formats. Some content that appears
in print may not be available in electronic books.

Cover image: iStock File #7646055 © Fertnig

Set in 9/12 pt Palatino by Toppan Best-set Premedia Limited

1 2014

Contents

Preface, vii

Acknowledgements, viii

Preface

Paediatrics is a rapidly evolving field of medicine, particularly in the sub-specialties. This makes it difficult for trainees, junior doctors and allied health professionals to keep up with new developments.

This book aims to provide problem-orientated clinical scenarios in paediatric gastroenterology, hepatology and nutrition, and is designed to make initial assessment, management and referral of children easy to follow.

The book is up to date with current practice, user friendly, with links to the latest guidance, protocols and information, and should be a popular book no trainee doctor should be without.

We hope you enjoy using it and that it will help you improve how you manage children with these specialist conditions.

Acknowledgements

Dr Indra van Mourik, Consultant Hepatologist, The Liver Unit, Birmingham Children's Hospital, Birmingham, UK

Sara Clark, Senior Dietitian, The Liver Unit, Birmingham Children's Hospital, Birmingham, UK

Simon Fraser, Nutrition Pharmacist, Royal Hospital for Sick Children, Glasgow, UK

Avril Smith, Gastrostomy Nurse Specialist, Royal Hospital for Sick Children, Glasgow, UK

Guftar Sheikh, Consultant Endocrinologist, Royal Hospital for Sick Children, Glasgow, UK

Gastroenterology

Abdominal symptoms are often non-specific, with a wide differential diagnosis. We aim to provide a framework for evaluation, with information for both common and important rare conditions. A multidisciplinary model of care supports optimal management and outcomes. Specialist nursing, dietetics and psychology are central to supporting therapy, especially in chronic illness. Specialist advice and management for rare or complex problems are important, as is recognising non-gastrointestinal illness and conditions requiring surgical intervention, often provided through a defined network of units with pathways for referral, and shared-care with community and hospital teams.

Practical Approach to Paediatric Gastroenterology, Hepatology and Nutrition, First Edition.
Deirdre Kelly, Ronald Bremner, Jane Hartley, and Diana Flynn.
© 2014 John Wiley & Sons, Ltd. Published 2014 by John Wiley & Sons, Ltd.

It can be difficult to distinguish between 'normal' colic and pathological conditions.

Infantile colic is common in the first months of life. Babies scream, draw up their knees and experience severe pain. Episodes may last up to 3 hours and occur several times per week. Causes are listed in Table 1.1.

Pathological pain from any site may be interpreted as abdominal in origin, e.g. corneal abrasion, renal tract obstruction, bony fracture.

Investigations

Normal results from screening blood tests can help reassure that underlying renal, liver or metabolic diseases are unlikely.
- FBC, renal, liver and bone biochemistry, blood gases
- Urine analysis and culture
- Plain abdominal radiograph: volvulus in the ill child or with bilious vomiting
- Abdominal ultrasound scan: when intussusception suspected
- Barium swallow and follow to the duodenal–jejunal flexure: to exclude malrotation
- Endoscopy is rarely indicated

Management

In the absence of other obvious cause, a time-limited trial of hypoallergenic feed can be useful to exclude milk allergy/intolerance (see Chapter 12), and antacid therapy can be used if there is acid reflux-related oesophagitis. Most often, colic settles within a few weeks or with changes in routine.

Practical Approach to Paediatric Gastroenterology, Hepatology and Nutrition, First Edition.
Deirdre Kelly, Ronald Bremner, Jane Hartley, and Diana Flynn.
© 2014 John Wiley & Sons, Ltd. Published 2014 by John Wiley & Sons, Ltd.

Table 1.1 Causes, cardinal signs and diagnostic investigations in a child with abdominal pain

Causes	Cardinal features	Diagnostic test
Infantile colic	No abnormal findings	None
Gastro-oesophageal reflux	Regurgitation, back arching	Trial of acid suppression
		Oesophageal (+gastric) pH probe
		Oesophageal impedance study
		Endoscopy and histology
Milk or soya allergy/intolerance	Diarrhoea, rashes	See Chapter 12
Gastroenteritis	Watery stools, fever	Stool virology/microbiology
Constipation	Straining, hard stool, retentive behaviour	See Chapter 14
Urinary tract infection	Fever, pyuria	Urine dipstick test for leukocytes and nitrites, or microscopy
		Microbial culture
Intussusception	Ill child, red currant jelly stools (late sign)	Fluoroscopy with air enema reduction
	Blood on digital rectal examination	
Volvulus	Distension, bilious vomiting	Abdominal radiograph
Incarcerated hernia	Tender groin swelling	Ultrasonography

Table 1.1 (*Continued*)

Causes	Cardinal features	Diagnostic test
Testicular torsion	Scrotum swollen and/or discoloured and/or tender	Ultrasonography
Hirschsprung's disease	Delayed passage of meconium, ribbon stools	Full thickness rectal biopsy
Renal pelviceal/ureteric obstruction	Recurrent urinary tract infection, episodic pain	Ultrasonography
Metabolic disease (e.g. Reye's syndrome, MCADD)	Acidosis, encephalopathy	Blood gases, glucose, ammonia, lactate, serum amino acids, urine amino and organic acids, acyl carnitines

MCADD, medium-chain acyl-CoA dehydrogenase deficiency.

Red flags: When colic is concerning

- Abdominal distension (see Chapter 6)
- Faltering growth: feeding problem (see Chapters 37, 38 and 39) or malabsorption (see Chapter 9)
- Abnormal developmental progress: severe oesophagitis more likely, underlying metabolic disorder

The child with abdominal pain

CHAPTER 2

Abdominal pain is common in school-aged children and is rarely organic.

History

- Duration and location [right upper quadrant pain in hepatitis, Gilbert's syndrome and non-alcoholic steatohepatitis (NASH)]
- Associated symptoms: vomiting, dyspepsia, diarrhoea, fever, groin pain, urinary symptoms
- Blood in stool
- Vaginal discharge
- Foreign travel
- Gynaecological and sexual history
- Family history: inflammatory bowel disease, coeliac disease, migraine, irritable bowel syndrome, gallstones, pancreatitis

Investigations

- Urinalysis: haematuria in renal stones, pyuria in urinary tract infection
- Urine microscopy, culture, sensitivities
- Blood tests: blood glucose, FBC, renal function, liver function, inflammatory markers, amylase, cholesterol, triglycerides
- Other blood tests if indicated, e.g. paracetamol levels, thyroid function tests
- Stool samples if diarrhoea: microscopy, culture, sensitivity, ova, cysts, parasites

Practical Approach to Paediatric Gastroenterology, Hepatology and Nutrition, First Edition.
Deirdre Kelly, Ronald Bremner, Jane Hartley, and Diana Flynn.
© 2014 John Wiley & Sons, Ltd. Published 2014 by John Wiley & Sons, Ltd.

- Abdominal imaging:
  - Abdominal X-ray, e.g. if looking for obstruction
  - Chest X-ray, e.g. for pneumonia or air under the diaphragm
  - Ultrasound scan of the abdomen, kidneys, pelvis (females) and testes (males)
  - CT scan may also be appropriate, especially if there is a mass, trauma, jaundice or pancreatitis
- Endoscopy: will depend upon preliminary findings and history; in the absence of any abnormality on blood screen and imaging, negative endoscopy is very likely

Causes

Well child

- Functional bowel disease: recurrent abdominal pain of childhood, abdominal migraine
- Lactose intolerance: worse with dairy products (ice cream and chocolate are high lactose)
- Gastro-oesophageal reflux ± oesophagitis: dyspepsia, epigastric pain, regurgitation
- Constipation: hard, infrequent stools, soiling
- Renal pelvic/ureteric obstruction: intermittent colicky loin pain
- Coeliac disease: variable association with iron deficiency, diarrhoea, oral ampthous ulceration
- Food allergy (see Chapter 12)
- NASH: associated with obesity and metabolic syndrome

Febrile child

- Gastroenteritis (bacterial or viral)
- Mesenteric adenitis
- Urinary tract infection (lower abdominal pain, loin pain – suggests pyleonephritis)
- Pneumonia
- Inflammatory bowel disease
- Liver abscess

The ill child

- Diabetic ketoacidosis: check urine for glucose, blood gases
- Mesenteric lymphadenitis: fever, often with associated tonsillitis or pharyngitis
- Peptic ulcer disease: sharp epigastric pain after meals
- Hepatitis: raised liver transaminases ± jaundice; see Chapter 21

- Pancreatitis: high amylase, bilirubin and transaminases may be raised
- Ultrasound: biliary dilatation may be seen in acute pancreatitis
- DNA: *PRSS1* mutations in familial pancreatitis, raised serum amylase and lipase
- Sickle cell anaemia/crisis: blood film shows sickle cells
- Henoch–Schönlein purpura: characteristic vasculitic rash, haematuria or proteinuria
- Acute adrenal failure: hyponatraemia ± hyperkalaemia, check for inappropriate urinary sodium losses

Surgical causes

- Appendicitis: low-grade fever, central then right iliac fossa pain, unable to stand (psoas irritation), beware of atypical symptoms
- Bowel obstruction, e.g. intussusception, volvulus: bilious vomiting, abdominal distension, tenderness
- Trauma, e.g. haematoma, pancreatitis, liver trauma: may present several days after the event. Low haemoglobin, CT scan will identify liver laceration/pancreatic transection or liver abscesses
- Incarcerated hernia: groin or scrotal swelling/discolouration/pain
- Peritonitis: rigid abdomen or distension with tenderness
- Liver abscess: ultrasound – abscess(es) in liver, raised white cell count, blood culture or aspirate from the abscess may grow pathogen (most commonly *Streptococcus* or *Klebsiella*)
- Gallstones/cholecystitis: sickle cell on blood film, raised bilirubin if obstruction, abnormal transaminases, high amylase if the ampulla of Vater is affected, cholesterol or triglycerides may be high, ultrasound – acoustic shadow (Figure 2.1), biliary dilatation if the gallstone is causing obstruction
- Testicular torsion: scrotal swelling, tenderness, discolouration
- Ureteric calculi: colicky pain, macro- or micro-scopic haematuria

Gynaecological causes

- Dysmenorrhoea or endometriosis: prior and/or during menstrual bleed
- Mittelschmerz: mid-cycle colicky pain
- Pelvic inflammatory disease: fever variable

Obstetric causes

- Ectopic pregnancy: sudden onset with shock or peritonism
- Ovarian cyst rupture/torsion
- Miscarriage/abortion/retained foetal products

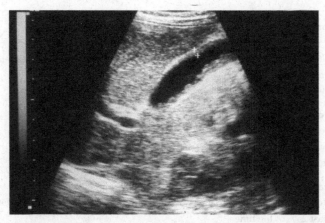

Figure 2.1 Ultrasound scan appearance of gallstones with acoustic shadows. The gallbladder wall (marked with crosses) is irregular and thick, consistent with chronic cholecystitis.

Drugs/toxins
- Paracetamol overdose
- Iron overdose
- Venoms: spider bite, scorpion sting
- Soap ingestion
- Erythromycin

Referred pain
- Usually musculoskeletal: examine for scoliosis, joint tenderness

Rare causes
- Angioneurotic oedema: episodic, rash or facial/lip swelling – allergy/immunology referral
- Familial Mediterranean fever or systemic lupus erythematosis: episodic fever and raised inflammatory markers with extra-intestinal symptoms – rheumatology referral
- Acute intermittent porphyria: episodic, send urine for porphyrins during an attack
- Peptic ulcer disease – often associated with *Helicobacter pylori* infection

Information: Rome III criteria for functional bowel diseases

- No evidence of an inflammatory, anatomical, metabolic or neoplastic process
- Symptoms: at least once a week for at least 2 months before diagnosis

Functional dyspepsia
- Persistent or recurrent pain or discomfort above the umbilicus
- Not relieved by defecation or associated with the onset of a change in stool frequency or stool form

Irritable bowel syndrome
Abdominal discomfort or pain associated with two or more of the following at least 25% of the time:
- Improved with defecation
- Onset associated with a change in frequency of stool
- Onset associated with a change in form (appearance) of stool

Functional abdominal pain
- Episodic or continuous abdominal pain
- Insufficient criteria for other functional gastrointestinal disorders

Functional abdominal pain syndrome
- Must include: functional abdominal pain at least 25% of the time and either some loss of daily functioning or additional somatic symptoms such as headache, limb pain or difficulty in sleeping

Information: Abdominal migraine

Criteria:
- Two or more times in the preceding 12 months
- Paroxysmal episodes of intense peri-umbilical pain lasting >1 hour
- Intervening periods of usual health lasting weeks to months
- Pain interferes with normal activities
- Pain is associated with two or more of the following:
  - Anorexia
  - Nausea
  - Vomiting
  - Headache
  - Photophobia
  - Pallor

Red flags: When to be concerned about abdominal pain

- Unintentional weight loss
- Growth failure or slowing
- Unexplained fever
- Chronic severe diarrhoea or significant vomiting
- Gastrointestinal bleeding
- Family history of inflammatory bowel disease
- Persistent chronic right iliac fossa or right upper quadrant pain
- Recurrent pancreatitis: consider hereditary pancreatitis or lipidaemia

---

Information: Gallstones

Associated with:
- Haemolysis
- Prematurity
- Cystic fibrosis
- Down's syndrome
- Bone marrow and cardiac transplantation
- Childhood cancer
- Spinal surgery/injury
- Hepatobiliary trauma
- Selective IgA deficiency
- Dystrophia myotonica
- Chronic intestinal pseudo-obstruction
- Cholestatic liver disease (especially progressive familial intrahepatic cholestasis)
- Congenital anomalies

  There is a bimodal incidence with initial peaks in infancy and adolescence; more common in females.

Presentation
- In infancy: poor feeding, vomiting and jaundice
- In older children: right upper quadrant or epigastric pain, nausea, vomiting and obstructive jaundice

Diagnosis
- Stones cast acoustic shadow on ultrasound and a thick-walled gallbladder (see Figure 2.1)

(Continued)

Outcome
- Infants: gallstones may resolve
- Older children: resolution is unlikely
- Surgery is only required if symptomatic or there is bile duct dilatation
- Laparoscopic cholecystectomy is advisable

Management

Functional abdominal pain
- Reassurance that there is no evidence of organic pathology
- Significant persistent symptoms require multidisciplinary input with a family-based holistic approach

Medications
- Functional abdominal symptoms respond poorly to acid reduction therapy or antispasmodics
- Peppermint oil (one or two capsules three times daily) is most likely to be effective
- Mebeverine hydrochloride: 25 mg three times daily (age 3–4 years); 50 mg three times daily (age 4–8 years); 100 mg three times daily (age 8–10 years); 135–150 mg three times daily (age over 10 years)
- Dicycloverine hydrochloride: 5–10 mg before feeds (age 6 months– 2 years); 10–20 mg three times daily (over age 2 years)
- Hyoscine butylbromide: 0.5 mg/kg, max. 5 mg three times daily (age 1 month–2 years); 5 mg three times daily (2–5 years); 10–20 mg three times daily (over 5 years)
- Abdominal migraine can be prevented or ameliorated by using a serotonin 2A receptor antagonist, pizotifen 0.25–0.5 mg twice or three times daily

Dietary management
Food allergy and intolerance is common in small children, and dietary manipulation is often attempted by families prior to seeking advice from health professionals. In practice, this is rarely effective and puts children at risk of nutrient deficiency (e.g. dairy exclusion and suboptimal calcium intake).

A careful history will identify those with food allergy or intolerance (see Chapter 12). Lactose intolerance is common in Asian and Afro-Caribbean populations. There is little evidence that functional abdominal pain improves with a lactose-free diet in either lactase-deficient or -sufficient children.

Probiotics and prebiotics have not been shown to be effective, though do no harm.

Psychological management

Functional abdominal pain may stem from learned-behaviour responses to environmental and social stimuli that interact with the child's experience of physical illness. This hypothesis is supported by psychological studies showing altered subliminal responsiveness to pain- and stress-related cues, and that maternal anxiety is a predictor. Psychological interventions, including family therapy, hypnotherapy and cognitive behavioural therapy, are effective in reducing the severity and duration of symptoms, and improving school attendance.

Gallstones

- Ursodeoxycholic acid 10–20 mg/kg/day with fat-soluble vitamins if there is obstructive jaundice
- Biliary dilatation requires removal of the stone by endoscopic manipulation through the ampulla of Vater using endoscopic retrograde cholangiopancreatography (ERCP)
- Laparoscopic cholecystectomy only when acute inflammation has resolved

Liver abscess

- Drainage of abscess
- Antibiotics (antifungals in immunosuppressed patients or if there is no response to antibiotics without culture sensitivities)

Liver trauma

- Resuscitation, pain relief, identify other injuries
- Conservative management unless haemorrhage is uncontrolled and then surgical intervention

Further reading

Berger MY, Gietling MJ, Benninga MA. Chronic abdominal pain in children. *BMJ* 2007;334:997–1002

Brown CW, Werlin SL, Geenen JE, Schmalz M. The diagnostic and therapeutic role of endoscopic retrograde cholangiopancreatography in children. *J Pediatr Gastroenterol Nutr* 1993;17:19–23

Huertas-Ceballos A, Logan S, Bennett C, Macarthur C. Psychosocial interventions for recurrent abdominal pain (RAP) and irritable bowel syndrome (IBS) in childhood. *Cochrane Database Syst Rev* 2008;1:CD003014

Huertas-Ceballos A, Logan S, Bennett C, Macarthur C. Pharmacological interventions for recurrent abdominal pain (RAP) and irritable bowel syndrome (IBS) in childhood. *Cochrane Database Syst Rev* 2008;1:CD003017

Huertas-Ceballos A, Logan S, Bennett C, Macarthur C. Dietary interventions for recurrent abdominal pain (RAP) and irritable bowel syndrome (IBS) in childhood. *Cochrane Database Syst Rev* 2008;1:CD003019

Key web links

http://79.170.44.126/britishlivertrust.org.uk/home-2/liver
-information/liver-conditions/gallstones/

http://www.naspghan.org/user-assets/Documents/pdf/disease
Info/Pancreatitis-E.pdf

Classification of functional GI disorders: the Rome III Criteria: http://
www.romecriteria.org/criteriaEvidence-based Guidelines from
ESPGHAN and NASPGHAN for *Helicobacter pylori* infection in children: http://espghan.med.up.pt/position_papers/Koletzko_Evidence
_based_Guidelines_From_ESPGHAN_and_NASPGHAN_for
_Helicobacter_pylori_Infection_in_Children.pdf – accessed 3/8/13

The infant with vomiting

Around half of infants regurgitate, and this on its own is not significant. However, vomiting is the cardinal feature of many gastrointestinal, renal, metabolic or neurological diseases. Persistent, effortless vomiting or posseting are characteristic of gastro-oesophageal reflux, and this is associated with a wide range of conditions, adding to the difficulty in management.

Important features from history

- Acute onset: infectious or surgical causes
- Fever: infection
- Antenatal history: maternal infection, antenatal ultrasound scan findings
- Birth history: prematurity, resuscitation
- Assess frequency and feed volume, characterise any feeding difficulties, effect of any changes in formulae
- Weight loss: systemic disease more likely
- Oesophagitis symptoms, e.g. irritability, back arching, feed refusal, haematemesis
- Failure to growth: no weight gain 2 weeks after birth or dropping through centiles
- Neurological symptoms and developmental progress: consider metabolic disease
- Family history of bowel surgery: malrotation, hiatus hernia, Hirschsprung's disease

Practical Approach to Paediatric Gastroenterology, Hepatology and Nutrition, First Edition.
Deirdre Kelly, Ronald Bremner, Jane Hartley, and Diana Flynn.
© 2014 John Wiley & Sons, Ltd. Published 2014 by John Wiley & Sons, Ltd.

- Cough or frequent chest infections: recurrent aspiration, cystic fibrosis, tracheo-oesophageal fistula
- Stridor or apnoea: seek ENT review
- Eczema, diarrhoea, urticaria or family history of atopy: suggest possible food allergy

---

Red flags: What to look for in a vomiting infant

- Exclude infection
- Always consider raised intracranial pressure: bulging fontanelle, climbing head circumference centiles
- Be alert to factitious or induced illness

Causes

Neonate

- Overfeeding: usual intake is 150–200 mL/kg/day
- Gastro-oesophageal reflux ± cow's milk intolerance/allergy
- Bowel obstruction: duodenal web, small bowel atresia, volvulus, malrotation, Hirschsprung's disease, imperforate anus
- Infection: gastroenteritis, septicaemia, urinary tract infection, pneumonia, meningitis
- Neonatal abstinence syndrome: opiate or amphetamine withdrawal
- Intracranial bleed or injury: bulging fontanelle
- Inborn error of metabolism, e.g. urea cycle disorder, fructosaemia
- Congenital adrenal hyperplasia: abnormal serum electrolytes
- H-type tracheo-oesophageal fistula: cough, recurrent aspiration
- Upper airway or ENT anomaly: apnoea, cough, choking

Older infant

- Overfeeding: usual intake is 120–150 mL/kg/day
- Gastro-oesophageal reflux
- Pyloric stenosis: blood gas for alkalosis, ultrasound scan, refer to surgeon for test feed
- Cow's milk protein intolerance/allergy: trial of hypoallergenic feed, or maternal milk/soya restriction
- Infection: gastroenteritis, urinary tract, otitis media, pneumonia, meningitis, septicaemia
- Intracranial mass, bleed or head injury: consider CT scan
- Bowel obstruction: abdominal radiograph, refer to surgeon
- Testicular torsion: urgent referral to surgeon

- Intussusception: ultrasound scan, refer to surgeon, air enema reduction
- Ketoacidosis: blood sugar, blood gas for acidosis
- Appendicitis: fever and abdominal pain, ultrasound scan, refer to surgeon
- Cystinosis: hypophosphataemia, renal tubular leak

Screening investigations (see Algorithm 3.1)

- Blood pressure
- Urine dipstix: ketones, sugar
- Blood sugar
- Septic screen if febrile or unwell
- Blood gases ± metabolic disease screen: blood ammonia, serum amino acids, urine amino and organic acids
- Serum biochemistry: U&E, LFT, bone profile
- Abdominal radiograph if obstruction suspected
- Barium swallow and follow through to the duodenal–jejunal flexure to exclude malrotation

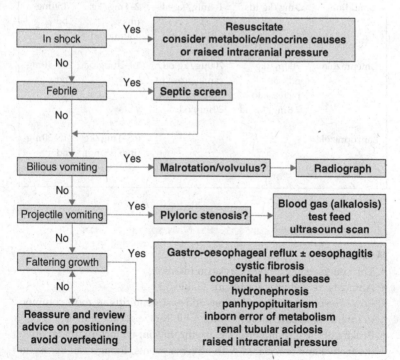

Algorithm 3.1 Investigation of vomiting in infants

Information: Tests for gastro-oesophageal reflux

Reflux events are common in normal infants, and not always symptomatic.
A barium meal is useful for malrotation or hiatus hernia, but not reflux.
Oesophageal pH (±impedance) probe studies (48–72 hours off antacids)
confirm acid reflux, but often do not alter management. Acid detection
greater than 10% of the time (the reflux index) indicates severe acid reflux,
which is associated with oesophagitis. False-negative results are common, as
are technical problems (misplaced or dislodged probe, inadequate symptom
diary, non-acid reflux events). Impedance studies provide more information
about non-acid events, but normative data are lacking.

Table 3.1 Doses for antacids in gastro-oesophageal reflux

	Neonate	Infant	1–12 years	Over 12 years
Ranitidine	2 mg/kg tds	1–3 mg/kg tds	2–4 mg/kg (max 150 mg) bd	150 mg bd
Omeprazole	700 µg/kg od, can increase to 2.8 mg/kg od	700 µg/kg od, can increase to 3 mg/kg (max 20 mg) od	10–20 mg od	20–40 mg od
Lanzoprazole	–	–	0.5–1 mg/kg (max 15 mg) od	15–30 mg od

Management of gastro-oesophageal reflux

Medication
- Thickeners, e.g. Carobel, Gaviscon infant
- Antacids: useful in oesophagitis (Table 3.1)
- Lower respiratory tract infections and gastroenteritis are more common in infants receiving proton pump inhibitors, e.g. omeprazole
- Prokinetics, e.g. domperidone, erythromycin, metoclopramide: often ineffective and associated with adverse events, though can be useful in difficult cases

Allied health professional
- Feed thickener or thickening formula
- Extensively hydrolysed formula or amino-acid formula (see Chapter 12)

Patient education

- Feed volume and frequency: feeding >150 mL/kg/day is likely to worsen reflux symptoms; smaller more frequent feeding can improve symptoms
- Positioning:
  - Although prone and left-lying positions are beneficial in reducing reflux in children younger than 6 months of age compared with supine or right-lying positions, these positions are associated with increased risk of sudden infant death syndrome
  - Elevating the head of the cot does not reduce reflux for infants in the supine position
  - An erect position for feeding and 20–30 minutes following feeds may reduce symptoms

Surgery
Fundoplication is indicated when symptoms are severe or life-threatening. It is a very effective operation with a low failure rate, but can have significant side-effects, including retching and dumping syndrome.

The neurodisabled infant
See Chapter 41

Outcome

- Even severe reflux is most often self-limiting and resolves as an infant is weaned and develops a more upright posture
- The risks for developing Barrett's oesophagus (metaplasia) and oesophageal carcinoma are not defined
- Cow's milk allergy (often associated with soya allergy): 85% resolve by 2 years old

---

Red flags: When to be concerned with vomiting

- Haematemesis: suggests severe erosive oesophagitis
- Bilious vomiting: volvulus, sepsis
- Faltering growth: investigate for other underlying conditions or feeding problem

Further reading

Huang RC, Forbes D, Davies MW. Feed thickener for newborn infants with gastro-oesophageal reflux. *Cochrane Database Syst Rev* 2002;Issue 3: CD003211

Vandenplas Y, Rudolph CD, Di Lorenzo C, *et al.* Pediatric gastroesophageal reflux clinical practice guidelines: joint recommendations of the North American Society for Pediatric Gastroenterology, Hepatology, and Nutrition (NASPGHAN) and the European Society for Pediatric Gastroenterology, Hepatology, and Nutrition (ESPGHAN). *J Pediatr Gastroenterol Nutr* 2009;49:498–547

Key web links

http://www.naspghan.org/user-assets/Documents/pdf/Position Papers/FINAL%20-%20JPGN%20GERD%20guideline.pdf
http://onlinelibrary.wiley.com/doi/10.1002/14651858.CD003211/full

The child with vomiting

CHAPTER 4

Important features from history

- Bilous vomiting is always pathological: consider bowel obstruction, malrotation or volvulus
- Associated neurological symptoms may alert to intracranial causes
- Morning vomiting without nausea is characteristic of a brain tumour
- Episodic vomiting with lethargy suggests cyclical vomiting syndrome, typically with ketosis

Differential diagnosis

- Always consider raised intracranial pressure
- Infection: gastroenteritis, urinary tract infection, upper respiratory tract infection, otitis media, pneumonia, meningitis, septicaemia
- Poisoning or drug-induced: alcohol, paracetamol, non-steroidals, digoxin, iron, antibiotics, theophylline, antiepileptics
- Gastro-oesophageal reflux ± oesophagitis
- Functional regurgitation
- Abdominal migraine: see Chapter 2, Information: Abdominal migraine
- Food allergy: associated lip/tongue tingling and/or swelling
- Cyclical vomiting syndrome: episodic and severe
- Faecal impaction
- Eosinophilic oesophagitis: often associated dysphagia, food impaction, atopy
- Crohn's disease: see Chapter 10
- Appendicitis: may present sub-acutely and/or with mass
- Pancreatitis: abdominal pain, may occur after blunt abdominal trauma
- Volvulus: abdominal pain, bilious vomiting, shock

Practical Approach to Paediatric Gastroenterology, Hepatology and Nutrition, First Edition.
Deirdre Kelly, Ronald Bremner, Jane Hartley, and Diana Flynn.
© 2014 John Wiley & Sons, Ltd. Published 2014 by John Wiley & Sons, Ltd.

- Achalasia: vomiting undigested food, dysphagia
- Ketoacidosis
- Head injury, brain tumour, intracranial bleeding or sinus venous thrombosis
- Hypertension
- Eating disorder: anorexia or bulimia, associated body image distortion
- Anxiety state, e.g. bullying, child abuse
- Factitious or induced illness

Investigations

- Blood pressure
- Urine dipstix: ketones, sugar
- Blood sugar
- Septic screen if febrile or unwell
- Blood gases ± metabolic disease screen: blood ammonia, serum amino acids, urine amino and organic acids
- Serum biochemistry: U&E, LFT, bone profile
- Amylase: beware of false positive after repeated vomiting (parotitis)
- Abdominal radiography: if bilious vomiting, for evidence of obstruction or volvulus
- Abdominal ultrasound: to examine the biliary tree, pancreas and renal tract
- Barium meal: to exclude malrotation

Management of cyclical vomiting

- Intravenous rehydration: often required if symptoms cannot be resolved quickly
- Drugs: early use of buccal antiemetics, e.g. ondansetron

Red flags: When to refer for specialist assessment ▶		
Symptom/finding	**Possible cause**	**Referral**
Haematemesis	Variceal or other upper GI bleed	Specialist centre
Bilious vomiting	Volvulus, obstruction	Surgeon
Abdominal distension/ tenderness	Peritonitis	Surgeon
Mass	See Chapter 13	Surgeon ± oncology
Altered consciousness	Raised intracranial pressure	Neurology
Papilloedema		Neurosurgeon ± oncology
New squint		
Early morning headache		
Distorted body image	Eating disorder	Psychiatrist
Lanugo		
Bradycardia		

Further reading

Vandenplas Y, Rudolph CD, Di Lorenzo C, *et al*. Pediatric gastroesophageal reflux clinical practice guidelines: joint recommendations of the North American Society for Pediatric Gastroenterology, Hepatology, and Nutrition (NASPGHAN) and the European Society for Pediatric Gastroenterology, Hepatology, and Nutrition (ESPGHAN). *J Pediatr Gastroenterol Nutr* 2009;49:498–547

Key web links

http://www.naspghan.org/user-assets/Documents/pdf/Position Papers/FINAL%20-%20JPGN%20GERD%20guideline.pdf
Family support and information for infantile reflux: http://www .livingwithreflux.org

Difficulty swallowing

Dysphagia refers to difficulty swallowing, either in the initial phases in the oropharyngeal cavity or in the oesophageal phase. Both result in feeding difficulties in infants.

Causes

- Oral/pharyngeal disorders, e.g. cleft palate, tongue tie (common, but rarely the cause)
- Neurological causes, e.g. pseudobulbar palsy
- Gastro-oesophageal reflux disease ± oesophagitis: infant and child
- Eosinophilic oesophagitis: infant and child (15–30% of cases with dysphagia)
- Tracheo-oesophageal fistula: infant with cough
- Achalasia: vomiting undigested food
- Crohn's disease: anorexia, oral or oesophageal involvement
- Foreign body, including nasogastric tube
- Oesophageal trauma: burn (e.g. heat, corrosive, caustic, radiation)
- Schatzki rings (lower oesophageal rings): barium swallow, endoscopy
- Oesophageal web
- Vascular ring
- Mediastinal mass: chest radiography and/or CT scan
- Drugs, e.g. doxorubicin, NSAIDs, antibiotics (e.g. clindamycin, doxycycline)
- Epidemolysis bullosa
- Anorexia nervosa
- Oesophageal candidiasis (Figure 5.1)

Practical Approach to Paediatric Gastroenterology, Hepatology and Nutrition, First Edition.
Deirdre Kelly, Ronald Bremner, Jane Hartley, and Diana Flynn.
© 2014 John Wiley & Sons, Ltd. Published 2014 by John Wiley & Sons, Ltd.

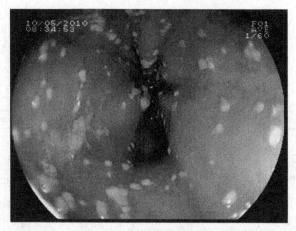

Figure 5.1 Endoscopic appearances of while papules in oesophageal candidiasis.

- Viral infection, e.g. herpes, CMV
- Chagas disease, megaoesophagus

Investigations (Algorithm 5.1)

- Videofluoroscopy
- Microlaryngoscopy if upper airway problems suspected
- Barium radiology: for stricture, compression, H-type tracheo-oesophageal fistula or achalasia
- Oesophageal manometry
- Flexible gastro-oesophagoscopy, with biopsies (multiple oesophageal levels)

Management

Ingested foreign bodies

- Batteries lodged in the oesophagus cause caustic burn and perforation within hours, especially with nickel/cadmium, and should be urgently removed by endoscopy. Batteries that remain in the stomach require retrieval
- Most other objects, even if sharp, pass harmlessly through the gut. Removal can cause oesophageal trauma
- Occasionally, a foreign body becomes impacted at the ligament of Trietz or the ileo-caecal valve and causes obstruction

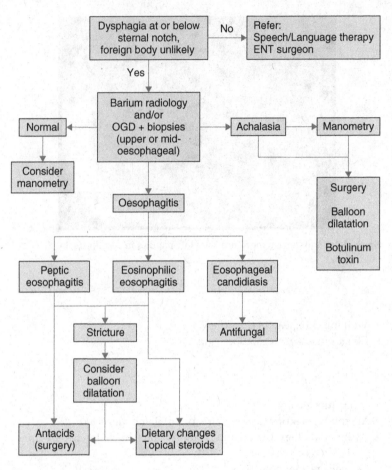

OGD, oesophagogastroduodenoscopy.

Algorithm 5.1 Assessment and management of swallowing difficulties

- Very rarely, an impacted foreign body lodged in the oesophagus erodes into other mediastinal structures. If suspected, surgical referral is required

Infant feeding disorder

Behavioural feeding problems are common, and often are not associated with an underlying medical or global developmental disorder, but are more common in children with other conditions, e.g. cerebral palsy, gastro-oesophageal reflux, cardiorespiratory illness or airway issues.

Early involvement of a Speech and Language Specialist and/or feeding psychologist for behavioural interventions is recommended. Encourage

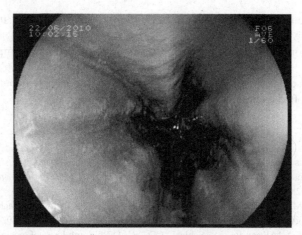

Figure 5.2 Eosinophilic oesophagitis with linear furrows.

a low-stress feeding environment and 'messy play'. An otherwise normal child can thrive on a surprisingly restricted diet.

Eosinophilic oesophagitis (EE)

The incidence of EE is 0.7 in 100 000 in the US. Most children have symptoms suggestive of gastro-oesophageal reflux disease (50–80%) or food impaction (20–50%). Typical endoscopic appearances are white plaques, ringed ('trachealised') oesophagus, linear furrows or a narrow oesophagus (Figure 5.2). Strictures occur. Because EE can be present in the presence of normal endoscopy, routine biopsies are essential, with >15 eosinophils seen in a high power field and/or eosinophilic microabscesses. Antireflux therapy is usually ineffective.

Elimination diets guided by allergy tests or complete food allergen exclusion are effective in 90% of cases. Use an elemental diet for 6–8 weeks, followed by staged food re-introduction. Relapse is common and a repeat may be required.

Corticosteroids are effective, but side-effects and relapse are common. Topical therapy is with oral flucticasone from a metered dose inhaler or viscous budenoside preparation. Azathioprine and other immune suppressants have been used in steroid-dependent disease.

Strictures should be balloon dilatated. Oesophageal tears are common, though rarely associated with perforation. Re-occurrence is usual.

Achalasia

Achalasia is characterised by non-relaxing muscle tone at the gastro-oesophageal sphincter and oesophageal dysmotility. The incidence is 0.2:100 000 in the UK children. The cause is unknown.

Calcium channel blockers have been used, but are usually ineffective.

Balloon dilations and injection of botulinum toxin provide temporary relief.

Open or laparoscopic Heller's myotomy has good long-term outcome, and is often combined with an antireflux operation.

Further reading

Liacouras CA, Furuta GT, Hirano I, et al. Eosinophilic esophagitis: updated consensus recommendations for children and adults. *J Allergy Clin Immunol* 2011;128:3–20.e6; quiz 21–22

Marlais M, Fishman JR, Fell JM, Haddad MJ, Rawat DJ. UK incidence of achalasia: an 11-year national epidemiological study. *Arch Dis Child* 2011;96(2):192–194

Prasad GA, Alexander JA, Schleck CD, et al. Epidemiology of eosinophilic esophagitis over three decades in Olmsted County, Minnesota. *Clin Gastroenterol Hepatol* 2009;7(10):1055–1061SSAT Patient Care Guideline: Esophageal achalasia. *J Gastrointest Surg* 2007;11:1210–1212

Key web links

http://www.fabed.co.uk (eosinophilic oesophagitis)
http://www.sts.org/patient-information/esophageal-surgery/
achalasia-and-esophageal-motility-disorders (achalasia)

Abdominal distension

The infant has a protuberant abdomen, with gaseous bowel and low abdominal wall muscle tone. After around 5 years of age, the abdomen should appear flat when the child is supine. Distension may be an associated symptom with several underlying pathologies, or secondary to a mass (see Chapters 13, 20 and 26).

Important features from history

- Onset: congenital, sudden or gradual, recent trauma
- Persistent or intermittent: worse in the evening?
- Vomiting: bilious?
- Bowel habit: frequency and character
- Blood in stool?
- Steatorrhoea
- Growth
- Past medical history: prematurity, jaundice or liver disease, infection, Crohn's disease
- Family history: Hirschsprung's disease, malrotation, coeliac disease, irritable bowel syndrome

---

Red flags: Abdominal distension

- Distension may be an early sign of necrotising enterocolitis in premature infants
- Early referral to a specialist surgical centre is often required
- Repeated episodes without surgical cause suggest chronic intestinal pseudo-obstruction

---

Practical Approach to Paediatric Gastroenterology, Hepatology and Nutrition, First Edition.
Deirdre Kelly, Ronald Bremner, Jane Hartley, and Diana Flynn.
© 2014 John Wiley & Sons, Ltd. Published 2014 by John Wiley & Sons, Ltd.

Differential diagnosis

- With mass: see Chapter 13:
  - Constipation with impaction
  - Malignancy: intra- or retro-peritoneal
  - Inflammatory mass, e.g. appendicitis, Crohn's disease, Meckel's diverticulitis
  - Renal/bladder obstruction
  - Choledochal cyst
  - Duplication cyst
- With organomegaly: see Chapters 20 and 26
- Aerophagia, usually less pronounced on morning waking
- Bezoar
- Constipation: faecaloma usually present
- Dysmotility: severe repeated episodes suggest chronic intestinal pseudo-obstruction
- Malabsorption ± enteropathy: see Chapters 9, 10 and 12
- Bacterial overgrowth: consider underlying malabsorption or dysmotility
- Stricture with partial obstruction
- Duplication cyst: stomach/duodenum/small bowel/colon
- Ascites and hepatic disease/tumours: see Chapters 20 and 26
- Necrotising enterocolitis
- Pancreatic pseudocyst
- Ovarian/pelvic tumour
- Hydro- or heamato-colpos
- Pregnancy/ectopic pregnancy

Investigations

- Abdominal ultrasound scan: organs, mass, ascites
- Plain radiography: if obstruction or perforation suspected
- CT scan for mass or after trauma, e.g. haemorrhage or pancreatic pseudocyst
- Barium radiology or magnetic resonance enterography if stricture or inflammatory bowel disease suspected
- Full thickness rectal biopsy: if Hirschsprung's suspected
- Urine or serum beta-human chorionic gonadotrophin (β-hCG): if pregnancy suspected

Management of bacterial overgrowth
(see Chapter 46)

If asymptomatic, no treatment is required. If associated with malabsorption or D-lactic acidosis, then treat with antibiotics. Non-absorbed oral antibiotics are often used in children with short-gut syndrome, e.g. gentamicin, neomycin, colomycin.

Key web link

The International Foundation for Functional Gastrointestinal Disorders: http://www.iffgd.org/

The infant with acute diarrhoea

CHAPTER 7

Diarrhoea is commonly caused by infectious gastroenteritis. It is a non-specific symptom in infants and older children, requiring a high index of suspicion for others diseases, especially septicaemia and meningitis.

Infants in developing nations may have repeated infectious diarrhoeal episodes and a secondary malabsorptive state, leaving them more vulnerable to malnutrition and further infections.

Non-infective acute diarrhoea may represent the effect of exposure to an allergen or sugar malabsorption (see Chapters 10 and 12).

Red flag: Risk of acute diarrhoea in infants
Infants are susceptible to dehydration, with a relative high body surface area for mass, raising insensible losses, and poor urinary concentrating ability.

Causes

- Infections (remember endemic illnesses after return from foreign travel):
  - Viruses: rotavirus, norovirus, adenovirus type 40/41, calicvirus, astrovirus
  - Bacteria: *Camplylobacter*, *Escherichia coli*, *Salmonella*, *Shigella*, cholera
  - Since 50% of neonates and young infants are colonised with Clostridium difficile, symptomatic disease is unlikely in children younger than 12 months
  - Parasites: *Cryptosporidium*, *Giardia*, *Entamoeba*

Practical Approach to Paediatric Gastroenterology, Hepatology and Nutrition, First Edition.
Deirdre Kelly, Ronald Bremner, Jane Hartley, and Diana Flynn.

- Drugs: laxatives
- Food additives, e.g. sorbitol in medications
- Food allergy or cow's milk protein intolerance
- Neonatal abstinence syndrome, e.g. opiate or amphetamine withdrawal

---

Red flags: When to consider diagnoses other than gastroenteritis

Not gastroenteritis if:
- Fever >38° (<3 months), >39° (>3 months)
- Bulging fontanelle, neck stiffness, altered consciousness
- Non-blanching rash
- Bilious vomiting
- Abdominal distension, with tenderness

Be concerned about:
- Repeated episodes: consider immune deficiency or other enteropathy
- Abdominal distension: see Chapter 6
- Diarrhoea persisting for >2 weeks, refer to specialist centre

---

Management

Fluid management
- If shock, IV fluids may be required (see Chapter 8)
- Start with 57 mL/kg oral rehydration solution (ORS) after each large watery stool (especially in infants <6 months or with low birth weight)
- If dehydration recurs, start ORS again

Early feeding reduces diarrhoea duration and improves nutritional outcome. Breast-fed infants should continue breast-feeding though their rehydration phase, and formula-fed infants returned to full-strength milk as soon as rehydration is complete, i.e. within a few hours. Normal diet should be re-introduced once rehydration is complete.

There is no evidence for regrading with diluted milk feeds in a normal child with acute gastroenteritis.

Rotavirus causes transient lactose intolerance. If there is recurrent diarrhoea upon milk re-introduction, give a lactose-free diet for a short period (usually <6 weeks).

Medication
- Antidiarrhoeal agents are not required
- Antiemetics may be used as an adjunct to oral rehydration therapy, e.g. ondansetron

- Antibiotics are indicated for *Salmonella* enteritis in infants younger than 6 months, and the malnourished or immunocompromised
- Seek expert microbiology advice before prescribing antibiotics in infants who have been abroad recently

Prevention

Breast-feeding reduces the incidence of diarrhoeal illness in both developing and developed countries.

Hygiene and good food preparation practices are central to reducing infection. Children should not attend childcare facilities for at least 48 hours after the last episode of infectious diarrhoea or vomiting. Towels should not be shared.

Rotavirus vaccines reduce severe illness and hospitalisation rates.

Further reading

Guarino A, Albano F, Ashkenazi S, *et al*. ESPGHAN/ESPID evidence-based guidelines for the management of acute gastroenteritis in children in Europe. *J Pediatr Gastroenterol Nutr* 2008;46:619–621

Madhi SA, Cunliffe NA, Steele D, Witte D, Kirsten M, Louw C. Effect of human rotavirus vaccine on severe diarrhea in African infants. *N Engl J Med* 2010;362:289–298

Key web link

NICE Clinical Guideline: Diarrhoea and vomiting caused by gastroenteritis in children under 5 http://www.nice.org.uk/cg84

The child with acute diarrhoea

Acute diarrhoea is common in children under 5 years. It is transient and caused by viral gastroenteritis, and management is supportive. Morbidity is worse in infants (see Chapter 7), those with malnutrition or other medical conditions, such as renal disease or short gut syndrome. Mortality is high in the under 5 year olds in developing nations with a high prevalence malnutrition and inadequate access to safe drinking water, causing almost 2 million child deaths per year, which represents almost one in five of all deaths in this age group. Oral rehydration solution (ORS) has reduced mortality by almost 50% since the 1970s. The UK formulation of ORS contains less sodium (see Information: Oral rehydration solution salt content), as severe sodium deficiency is less common.

Important features from history

- Duration
- Vomiting
- Stool frequency and character: blood present?
- Fluid and dietary intake
- Travel
- Contact with illness
- Exposure to animals, e.g. petting zoo or children's farms
- Weight loss: look for a recent weight in the Child Health Record
- Urine output: *beware* – watery stool can be mistaken for urine
- Drugs: antibiotics, prokinetics, immunosuppressants
- Past history: a wide range of co-morbid conditions increase the severity of illness or affect the capacity to respond to dehydration

Practical Approach to Paediatric Gastroenterology, Hepatology and Nutrition, First Edition.
Deirdre Kelly, Ronald Bremner, Jane Hartley, and Diana Flynn.
© 2014 John Wiley & Sons, Ltd. Published 2014 by John Wiley & Sons, Ltd.

Clinical course

- Infectious diarrhoea usually lasts 5–7 days and resolves within 2 weeks
- Vomiting is commonly associated and lasts 2–3 days

Causes

- Viruses: rotavirus, norovirus, adenovirus type 40/41, calicvirus, astrovirus
- Bacteria: *Camplylobacter*, *Escherichia coli*, *Salmonella*, *Clostridium difficile* (especially after antibiotics), *Shigella*, cholera
- Parasites: *Cryptosporidium*, *Giardia*, *Entamoeba*
- Drugs: antacids, oral calcium or phosphate salts, methylxanthines
- Food additives: sorbitol, caffeine, monosodium glutamate
- Food allergy or intolerances

Assessment

- Clinical assessment of dehydration is difficult and often inaccurate
- If a recent accurate pre-illness weight is available, the fluid deficit can be estimated from the weight loss
- Red flag symptoms indicate a child at risk of progression to shock (see Information: Signs of dehydration)
- If shock is present, consider both severe dehydration and septicaemia
- Most children do not require serum or urine tests, as they are unlikely to be helpful in determining the degree of dehydration
- Some children with peritonism or meningitis present with diarrhoea (and/or vomiting), but often there are other clinical features to alert the clinician to this diagnosis

Information: Comparison of clinical features in mild/moderate dehydration and hypovolaemic shock in severe dehydration

Assessing dehydration accurately at the bedside is difficult, but clinical signs of shock warn of severe illness. Frequent review is required to anticipate deterioration.

	Dehydration	Shock
Symptoms	Irritable/lethargic	Decreased consciousness
Signs	Skin colour unchanged	Pale or mottled skin
	Warm extremities	Cold extremities
	Normal peripheral pulses	Weak peripheral pulses
Observations	Normal capillary return	Delayed capillary return (>2 seconds)
	Normal blood pressure	Low blood pressure (pre-morbid sign)

Fluid management

Fluid management

- Encourage oral fluid intake, avoid fruit juices and carbonated drinks (high osmolality and low sodium)
- Offer ORS as a supplemental fluid for those at risk of dehydration
- In dehydration without shock, give 50 mL/kg ORS over 4 hours
- IV fluids: if no improvement, vomiting of ORS by mouth or nasogastric tube
- Clinical practice guidelines vary for IV fluid rehydration: most recommend an isotonic solution, e.g. 0.9% saline or Hartmann's, with a maintenance volume, plus an additional 50–100 mL/kg/day depending on the severity of fluid depletion
- Glucose may be required in a small child or after prolonged starvation, e.g. 5% dextrose in 0.9% saline

Risks of IV fluid rehydration include hyponatraemia (leading to seizures), raised intracranial pressure and (rarely) death. Ensure sufficient electrolyte content in IV rehydration fluids. Monitor clinical state and plasma electrolytes at baseline and during therapy.

In hypernatraemic dehydration, correction of fluid and electrolyte imbalance should take place over 24–48 hours. Oral fluids, e.g. ORS, should be continued during IV rehydration, and should be included in the fluid balance assessment. If tolerated, stop IV fluids and continue oral rehydration.

Introduce normal milk and diet after rehydration, but avoid fruit juices and carbonated drinks until diarrhoea resolves. Children with medical conditions may need regrading onto a normal diet if relapse is to be avoided.

Medication

- Antidiarrhoeal agents are not required
- Antibiotics are not routinely required, except in children with suspected or confirmed septicaemia, immunodeficiency, giardiasis or bacterial dysentery. Antibiotics may prolong carrier state in *Salmonella* infection and increase the risk of the haemolytic uraemic syndrome in *E. coli* infection
- Ondansetron, a 5-HT$_3$ receptor antagonist, reduces vomiting in children with gastroenteritis, leading to fewer failing oral rehydration and thus reducing the requirement for IV fluids and hospitalisation

Other therapies
- Probiotics reduce the duration of diarrhoea, with efficacy for *Lactobacillus casei* GG in rotavirus infections
- Zinc supplementation reduces the duration of diarrhoea and the incidence of prolonged diarrhoea (over 7 days) in malnourished children with acute gastroenteritis

---

Information: Oral rehydration solution salt content (mmol/L)

	UK formula	WHO formula
Sodium	60	75
Potassium	20	20
Chloride	60	65
Citrate	10	10
Glucose	90	75

Further reading

Allen SJ, Martinez EG, Gregorio GV, Dans LF. Probiotics for treating acute infectious diarrhoea. Cochrane Database Syst Rev 2010;Issue 11:CD003048

Freedman SB, Adler M, Seshadri R, Powell EC. Oral ondansetron for gastroenteritis in a pediatric emergency department. *N Engl J Med* 2006;354:1698–1705

Hartling L, Bellemare S, Wiebe N, Russell KF, Klassen TP, Craig WR. Oral versus intravenous rehydration for treating dehydration due to gastroenteritis in children. Cochrane Database Syst Rev 2006;Issue 3:CD004390

Patro B, Golicki D, Szajewska H. Meta-analysis: zinc supplementation for acute gastroenteritis in children. *Aliment Pharmacol Ther* 2008;28:713–723

Key web link

NICE Clinical Guideline: Diarrhoea and vomiting caused by gastroenteritis in children under 5 http://www.nice.org.uk/cg84

The infant with chronic diarrhoea

Chronic diarrhoea in an infant is defined as diarrhoea that persists for >2 weeks. Many infants with malabsorption, infection or underlying systemic disease have faltering growth. Food allergy is over-diagnosed and over-treated.

Important features from history

- Onset: immediate onset at birth? at weaning? after first exposure to specific foods?
- Stool volume and character: blood in stool suggests colitis
- Dietary history: previous milk formulae, timing and details of weaning
- Family history and consanguinity
- Polyhydramnios: suggests microvillous inclusion disease or sodium/chloride transporter defect
- Neonatal history, e.g. prematurity and necrotising enterocolitis
- Medical history and drug exposure, e.g. congenital thyrotoxicosis
- Surgical history: gut length, ileo-caecal valve intact, whole colon, gastrostomy
- Growth trajectory
- Travel history: infection exposure
- Skin rashes: perianal irritation, eczema (associated with immunodeficiency syndromes)

Practical Approach to Paediatric Gastroenterology, Hepatology and Nutrition, First Edition.
Deirdre Kelly, Ronald Bremner, Jane Hartley, and Diana Flynn.
© 2014 John Wiley & Sons, Ltd. Published 2014 by John Wiley & Sons, Ltd.

> **Information: Defining the type of diarrhoea helps direct the assessment of cases**
>
> - Osmotic diarrhoea:
>   - Stops on fasting within 24 hours
>   - Stool pH usually <5 (acid from fermented malabsorbed sugars)
>   - Low stool sodium (<70 mmol/l)
>   - High measured osmolality (often >400)
> - Secretorydiarrhoea:
> - Continues despite fasting
>   - Fasting stool pH usually >6
>   - High stool sodium (>70 mmol/L)
>   - High measured osmolality (often 280–320 mOsmol/L)
> - Osmolar gap: measured osmolality minus calculated osmolality ($[Na] + [K]) \times 2$
> - Protein-losing enteropathy: steatorrhoea, hypoalbuminaemia, raised stool alpha-1-antitrypsin levels, lymphopoenia and hypogammaglobulinaemia

Differential diagnosis (see Algorithm 9.1)

- Common:
  - Non-specific (functional diarrhoea), e.g. toddler diarrhoea
  - Post-infectious (transient) lactase deficiency
  - Cow's milk/soya protein intolerance
  - Coeliac disease (see Chapter 12)
  - Cystic fibrosis
  - Short bowel syndrome
  - Motility disorder, e.g. after gastroschisis repair
  - Infectious, e.g. *Cryptosporidium*, *Giardia*, *Entamoeba*
  - After chemotherapy or radiotherapy
  - Graft-versus-host disease
  - Drug side-effects
- Rare:
  - Primary or acquired immune deficiency: recurrent infection, skin rashes
  - Sucrase–isomaltase deficiency: watery diarrhoea onset at weaning
  - Infant-onset inflammatory bowel disease, e.g. interleukin (IL)-10 receptor deficiency
  - Secretory tumours, e.g. VIPoma: abdominal mass, abnormal gut hormone profile
  - Lymphangectasia: raised stool alpha-1-antitrypsin

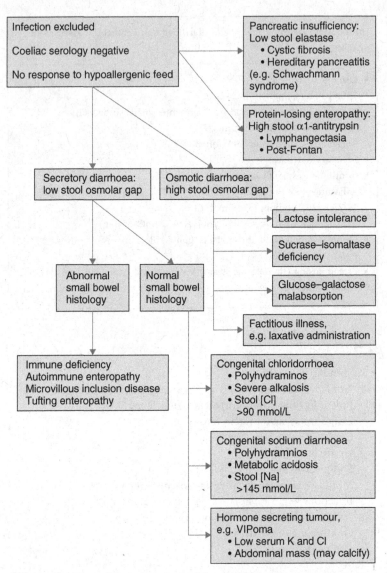

Algorithm 9.1 Biochemical assessment of chronic diarrhoea in infants

- Pancreatic insufficiency, e.g. Schwachmann syndrome (neutropoenia and skeletal abnormalities)
- Autoimmune enteropathy: antienterocyte antibody
- Abetalipoproteinaemia: acanthocytes on blood film
- Chlylomicron retention disease (Anderson's disease): typical small bowel histology
- Zinc deficiency: perianal and perioral skin rash
- Eosinophilic gastroenteritis: typical small bowel histology
- Intractable diarrhoea syndromes:
  - Congenital chloride diarrhoea
  - Congenital sodium diarrhoea
  - Glucose–galactose malabsorption
  - Microvillous inclusion disease
  - Tufting enteropathy
  - Trichohepatoenteric syndrome (phenotypic diarrhoea of infancy)

Toddler diarrhoea

This is a rapid transit, osmotic diarrhoea worsened by indigestable fruit sugars (or sorbitol), or an exaggerated gastrocolic reflex. It occurs after weaning or at the beginning of potty training. Stools often contain undigested food pieces.

Investigations
Stool samples for malabsorption and screening blood tests are normal.

Treatment
- Reduce fibre intake
- Avoid excessive fruit juices intake
- Loperamide

Outcome
Usually resolves by age 6 years.

Protein-losing enteropathy

May also have chylous ascites and/or chylothorax.

Causes
- Primary intestinal lymphangectasia:
  - Idiopathic
  - Turner's syndrome
  - Noonan's syndrome

- Secondary intestinal lymphangectasia:
  - Cardiac: post-Fontan procedure, constrictive pericarditis, cardiomyopathy
  - Obstructive: malrotation, tuberculosis, lymphoma, sarcoid
- Mucosal damage:
  - Infection: bacterial dysentery, *Giardia*, *Clostridium difficile*
  - Inflammatory: Crohn's disease, ulcerative colitis, necrotising enterocolitis, cow's milk protein intolerance, hypertrophic gastritis (Ménétrier's disease), eosinophilic gastroenteropathy, immune deficiency (e.g. common variable immune deficiency), graft-versus-host disease
  - Vasculitis: lupus, connective tissue disorders, Henoch-Schönlein purpura

Investigations
- Low immunoglobulins and lymphopoenia (from gut loss)
- Exclude cardiac, infectious or obstructive causes. Constrictive pericarditis may have an insidious onset and may be difficult to diagnose
- ^{99}Tc-labelled albumin scintigraphy, endoscopy and wireless capsule endoscopy to investigate lesion extent

Management
- High medium-chain triglyceride, low long-chain triglyceride diet
- Supplement fat-soluble vitamins (A/D/E/K)
- Transient symptomatic relief from albumin infusions (3–5 ml/kg 20% over 4–6 hours)
- Intractable cases require long-term parenteral nutrition. Refer to a specialist centre

Outcome
Some idiopathic cases improve with age. Segmental disease can be resected at surgery.

Investigations (screening tests in bold)

- **Blood count, renal, liver and bone biochemistry**
- Clotting studies: for vitamin K deficiency
- Blood gases: bicarbonate loss or electrolyte imbalance, e.g. potassium, chloride, lead to acidosis
- Stool analysis:
  - **Bacterial, viral and parasite examinations**
  - **Stool reducing sugars**
  - **Stool pH <5.5: suggests bacterial fermentation of undigested sugars**

- Stool fat analysis: steatocrit or microscopy for fat globules
- Elastase: for pancreatic exocrine function
- Faecal alpha-1-antitrypsin level: for protein loss
- **Coeliac serology**:
  - IgA tissue transglutaminase
  - Endomysial antibody
  - HLA-DQ2/DQ8
- Nutritional markers:
  - Vitamins A/D/E
  - Zinc, copper and selenium
  - Vitamin B_{12} and folate
  - Cholesterol and triglycerides
- Immune function work-up:
  - **Immunoglobulins A/G/M/E**
  - IgG subclasses
  - Functional antibody titres to vaccinations (tetanus, *Haemophilus*, *Pneumococcus*)
  - Lymphocyte subsets, including regulatory T-lymphocytes (CD 25+)
  - Neutrophil function: respiratory burst and migration
- Gut and vasoactive hormones:
  - Serum gastrin and vasointestinal peptide
  - Urinary catecholamines, e.g. VMA, HVA, dopamine
- Abdominal ultrasound scanning: for intra-abdominal or adrenal mass
- Barium follow-through: for stricture and web, and to assess transit, especially in a child with a history of necrotising enterocolitis; exclude gastro-colic fistula after gastrostomy
- Investigative dietary trials:
  - 48-hour fast: secretory diarrhoea?
  - Fructose-based diet: for glucose–galactose malabsorption
  - Lactose-free diet
  - Hypoallergenic diet
- Endoscopy:
  - Biopsy of duodenum for light and electron microscopy
  - Mucosal disaccharidase analysis
  - Microscopy and culture of duodenal juice
  - Sigmoidoscopy/colonoscopy
- Genetic defects in intractable diarrhoea:
  - Tufting enteropathy: *EpCAM*
  - Microvillous inclusion disease: *MYO5B*
  - Trichohepatoenteric syndrome (phenotypic diarrhoea): *TTC37*
  - Congenital chloride diarrhoea: *DRA*
  - Congenital sodium diarrhoea: *SPINT2*

Management

- Feed administration: use enteral tube feeding to maximise feed tolerance
- Dietary manipulation:
  - Extensively hydrolysed whey protein formulae (EHF) for malabsorption
  - Amino acid-based formulae: useful in allergy resistant to EHF
  - Medium-chain fatty acid formulae: for fat malabsorption
  - Pectin thickens and used as a pre-biotic: useful when a colon is present
  - Pancreatic enzyme replacement
- Parenteral nutrition: see Chapters 42–48
  - Nutritional rehabilitation during investigations and feed changes
- Drugs:
  - Loperamide: for rapid-transit or as an antisecretory agent
  - Colestyramine: for bile-salt malabsorption

Red flags: When to refer to specialist centre

- Watery diarrhoea since birth
- Severe and/or refractory faltering growth
- Secretory diarrhoea without obvious cause

Red flags: Pitfalls in managing chronic diarrhoea

- Watery stool can be easily mistaken for urine
- Functional disorders are very common and are not associated with growth failure or nutrient deficiency. However, misguided dietary restriction can reduce intake and result in growth impairment or specific nutrient deficiency
- Consider factitious or induced illness if diarrhoea is unexplained, e.g. laxative administration

The child with chronic diarrhoea

Chronic diarrhoea in a child is defined as the abnormal passage of three or more loose or liquid stools per day for >4 weeks, or a change in usual bowel habit to more loose or frequent stools. Associated weight loss, systemic illness or malabsorption is suggestive of a serious underlying cause.

Important features from history

- Onset
- Stool frequency and character
- Blood in stool
- Weight loss
- Growth trajectory
- Travel
- Previous gastroenteritis
- Dietary triggers
- Drug ingestion
- Family history

Differential diagnosis

- Common:
  - Irritable bowel syndrome
  - Coeliac disease (UK prevalence 1 in 100–200)
  - Food (or food additive) allergy or intolerance
  - Late-onset or post-infectious lactose intolerance
  - Infection: *Giardia*

Practical Approach to Paediatric Gastroenterology, Hepatology and Nutrition, First Edition.
Deirdre Kelly, Ronald Bremner, Jane Hartley, and Diana Flynn.

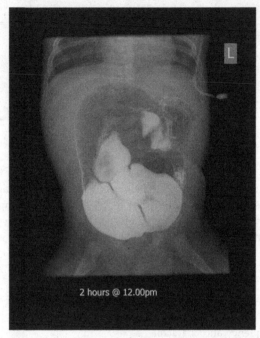

Figure 10.1 Barium radiology showing dilated small bowel loops in short gut syndrome, with stasis of luminal contents, predisposing to bacterial overgrowth.

- ○ Inflammatory bowel disease (UK incidence 5.6 per year per 100 000 children)
- ○ After chemotherapy or radiotherapy
- • Rare:
  - ○ Drug-related, e.g. non-steroidal anti-inflammatory drugs, mycophenolate mofetil
  - ○ Motility disorders, e.g. pseudo-obstruction
  - ○ Bacterial overgrowth, including the blind loop syndrome (Figure 10.1)
  - ○ Hyperthyroidism
  - ○ Hypoparathyroidism
  - ○ Addison's disease
  - ○ Hormone-secreting tumours, e.g. VIPoma
  - ○ Laxative abuse
  - ○ Primary bowel tumour
  - ○ Polyposis syndromes
  - ○ Lymphangectasia or other protein-losing enteropathy

Investigations

- Blood count, renal, liver and bone biochemistry
- Inflammatory markers, e.g. ESR, CRP
- Immunoglobulins A/G/M/E
- Specific IgE levels to food antigens: milk/soya/egg/wheat/nuts/ fish
- Coeliac serology:
  - IgA tissue transglutaminase
  - Endomysial antibody
  - HLA-DQ2/DQ8
- Stool analysis:
  - Bacterial, viral and parasite examinations
  - Calprotectin: a neutrophil protein stable in stool. Although specificity is suboptimal, a negative result reassures that inflammatory bowel disease is unlikely
- Small bowel imaging (Figure 10.2):
  - Magnetic enterography with oral and intravenous contrast
  - Barium meal and follow-through (± per-oral pneumocolon)
  - Ultrasound scanning: bowel wall thickness, increased vascularity, mass
- Investigative dietary trials:
  - Lactose-free diet
  - Hypoallergenic diet
  - Lactose/sucrose/fructose breath tests (poor sensitivity and specificity)
  - Endoscopy: oesophago-gastro-duodenoscopy and ileocolonoscopy with biopsies (Figure 10.3)

Red flags: Pitfalls in the diagnosis of diarrhoea

- Spurious diarrhoea in functional constipation with incomplete rectal emptying
- Anaemia, raised inflammatory markers and/or low serum albumin suggest inflammatory bowel disease
- Malnutrition is common in Crohn's disease, including deficiency of iron, vitamin B_{12}, vitamin D and zinc

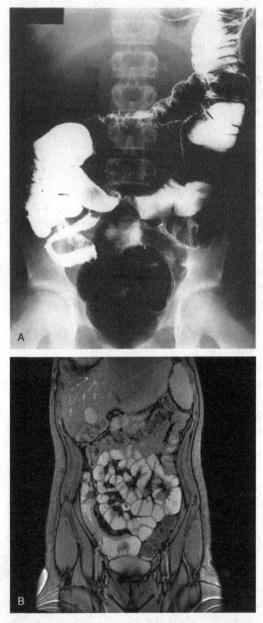

Figure 10.2 (A) Barium radiology showing bowel loop separation and 'rose-thorn' ulceration of the terminal ileum and right colon in Crohn's disease. (B) Magnetic resonance enterography provides imaging of the lumen, mucosa and bowel wall. A thick-walled narrow diseased segment in the right iliac fossa, with an area of pseudosacculation abutting the bladder (high signal from contrast in the lumen) and bowel loop separation with fat-wrapping (low signal).

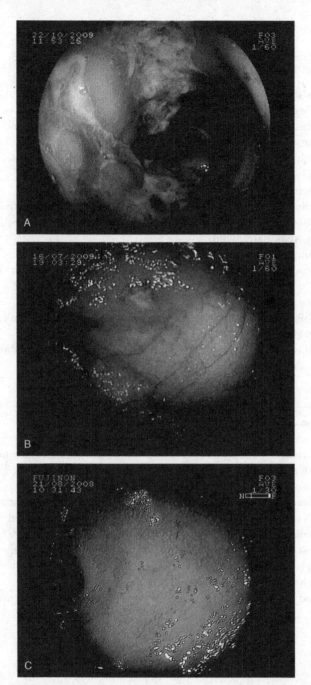

Figure 10.3 Endoscopic appearances of lesions in inflammatory bowel disease. (A,B) Crohn's disease deep linear 'snail-track' ulcers (A) or apthous ulcers (B). (C) Ulcerative colitis is typically diffusely red with bleeding and 'grains of salt' granularity.

Management

Crohn's disease (see Algorithm 10.1)

Inducing remission

- Exclusive enteral nutrition, for 6–8 weeks to induce remission:
  - Patient acceptance limits its use
  - Polymeric feeds are more palatable then elemental formulae
  - Nasogastric tube feeding can be a solution in some cases
- Systemic corticosteroids:
  - Administered parentally in severe disease, e.g. IV methyprednisolone 1–2 mg/kg (max 60 mg) per day or hydrocortisone 2 mg/kg (max 100 mg) qid
  - Supplemental nutrition is often required by NG tube
  - Specific nutrient deficiencies are common, e.g. iron, vitamin D, zinc

Disease relapse

- Exclusive enteral nutrition for 6–8 weeks and oral corticosteroids are both effective in 60–80% of cases
- Active perianal disease: metronidazole 7.5 mg/kg/dose tds and/or ciprofloxacin 5 mg/kg/dose bd

---

Information: Exclusive enteral nutrition liquid diet therapy

- Polymeric (whole protein) or elemental (amino acid) liquid diet formula with remission is usually attained within 1–2 weeks, is effective for luminal, oral and perianal disease
- Efficacy can be affected patient and parent choice, compliance, palatability
- Has added benefits of avoiding corticosteroid toxicity and improved nutritional status
- Most children need approximately 120% of estimated average energy requirement for age. This however needs to be adjusted according to individual needs and dietetic support is essential
- Food re-introduction over 1–3 weeks, dependent on patient symptoms

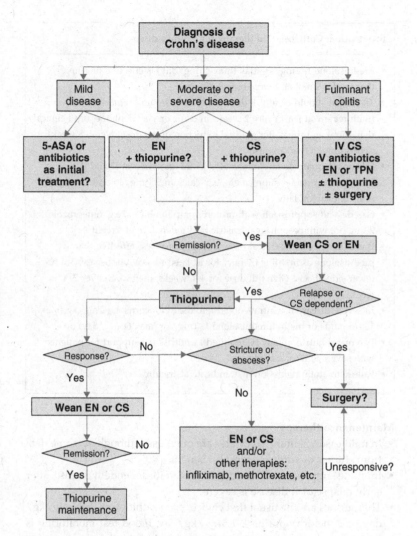

5-ASA, aminosalicylates; CS corticosteroids; EN, enteral nutrition.

Algorithm 10.1 Management of Crohn's disease

Information: Corticosteroid therapy for Crohn's disease

- Prednisolone 1–2 mg/kg/day (max 40 mg/day) is effective first-line therapy for small and large bowel disease
- Treatment should be at full dose for 2–4 weeks until remission achieved (with review at least every 2 weeks in clinic or via telephone, until clinical remission) and thereafter gradual reduction of the dose over 4–8 weeks depending on the response
- Ensure adequate dietary intake of calcium and vitamin D and if insufficient consider supplement, e.g. calcium 500 mg/colecalciferol 400 units one tablet daily
- Gastric acid suppression with proton pump inhibitors, e.g. omeprazole 20 mg od, with oesophageal, gastric or duodenal involvement
- Budesonide controlled ileal release 9 mg/day is less effective than prednisolone as first-line therapy for isolated ileo-caecal disease, but has fewer side-effects. Give full dose for 4–6 weeks, then wean over 2–4 weeks
- In severe disease use intravenous steroids: hydrocortisone 2 mg/kg (max 100 mg) qds or methylprednisolone 1–2 mg/kg (max 60 mg/day) od
- Parenteral nutrition may be required as nutritional support for patients with severe and/or complicated disease
- Failure to attain remission may indicate a stricture

Maintenance therapy
- In mild cases, 5-aminosalicylates are often used, though outcome data from studies of adults suggest no benefit
- Immune suppression is introduced in steroid-dependent disease, after early relapse or if disease is severe
- Thiopurines are the usual first choice, e.g. azathioprine 2–2.5 mg/kg/ day or 6-meracatopurine 1–1.5 mg/kg/day. Blood test monitoring is mandatory for bone marrow suppression. Metabolite measurements (6-thioguanine nucleotide and 6-methyl-mercaptopurine) are used to monitor compliance and risk of side-effects
- An alternative is methotrexate by subcutaneous injection (15 mg/m^2 weekly), with folic acid rescue, e.g. 5 mg po 6 days per week – not on the day of methrotrexate injection
- Antitumour necrosis factor antibodies, e.g. infliximab and adalimumab, are very effective in luminal and perianal disease that responds poorly to other treatments, although concerns about safety remain, with rare case reports of hepatosplenic lymphoma and severe infec-

tion. Most lymphomas have been in young men on concomitant immune suppression with azathioprine/6-mercaptopurine. These should be prescribed and supervised by a specialist

Surgery

Severe disease or disease unresponsive to second-line therapy should be discussed early with a surgeon with special expertise in inflammatory bowel disease. Fistulating perianal disease may respond to medical therapy combined with Seton drain insertion. Limited resections or stricturoplasty are preferred in luminal Crohn's disease, as repeated or large resections can result in short gut syndrome. In severe perianal or colonic disease, a diverting stoma can allow healing, although reversal may lead to relapse.

Future therapies

- New immunomodulators and biological therapies are being tested
- Autologous heamatopoetic stem cell transplantation is undergoing evaluation in adults
- Mesenchymal stem cell therapy offers theoretical advantages, with no requirement for pretransplant myeloablation or requirement for immune suppression

Ulcerative colitis

The majority (90%) of children with ulcerative colitis have pancolitis, <10% have left-sided colitis, 4% have disease confined to the rectum alone and 4% have rectal sparing.

Infective aetiology should be sought as this may co-exist with active disease, but in severe disease, immediate treatment with corticosteroids should not be delayed.

Acute severe colitis and/or toxic megacolon are life-threatening and should prompt urgent intervention. Second-line agents, e.g. ciclosporin, tacrolimus, infliximab, are potent immune suppressants with significant side-effect risks and should be managed by specialist centres.

Assessment of disease severity

- The paediatric ulcerative colitis activity (PUCAI) score (see Information: PUCAI score) combines clinical findings to give a numeric score for disease severity: remission <10; mild–moderate 10–60; severe: >65
- Fever, tachycardia, abdominal distension, abdominal tenderness, severe anaemia and hypoalbuminaemia suggest severe disease
- Abdominal radiograph for assessment of colonic dilatation (>4 cm diameter)

Information: PUCAI score

Item	Score
1. Abdominal pain	
None	0
Can be ignored	5
Cannot be ignored	10
2. Rectal bleeding	
None	0
Small amount only; in <50% of stools	10
Small amount with most stools	20
Large amount (>50% of the stool content)	30
3. Stool consistency of most stools	
Formed	0
Partially formed	5
Completely unformed	10
4. Number of stools per 24 hours	
0–2	0
3–5	5
6–8	10
>8	15
5. Nocturnal stools	
No	0
Yes	10
6. Activity level	
No limitation	0
Occasional limitation	5
Severe restriction	10

Treatment
- Severe colitis requires referral to a specialist centre (see Algorithm 10.2)
- Treatment with 5-aminosalicylates (ASAs) for mild/moderate disease:
  - Mesalazine 60–100 mg/kg/day (up to 4.8 g/day) for active colitis
  - Mesalazine 30–100 mg/kg/day up to 4.8 g/day for maintenance of quiescent or inactive colonic disease
  - Sulphasalazine 50–80 mg/kg/day up to 4 g/day for active colitis
  - Sulphasalazine 25–80 mg/kg/day up to 4 g/day for maintenance of quiescent or inactive disease

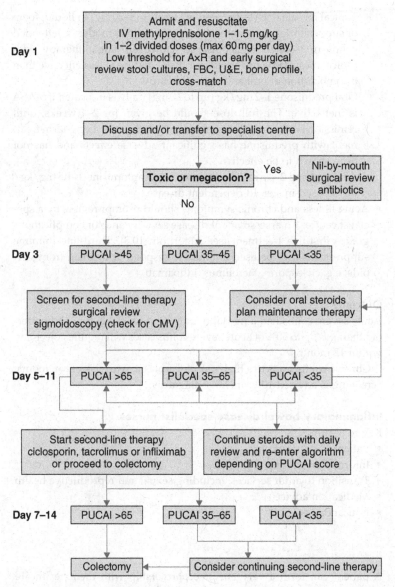

Day 1

Admit and resuscitate
IV methylprednisolone 1–1.5 mg/kg
in 1–2 divided doses (max 60 mg per day)
Low threshold for AxR and early surgical
review stool cultures, FBC, U&E, bone profile,
cross-match

Discuss and/or transfer to specialist centre

Toxic or megacolon? — Yes → Nil-by-mouth surgical review antibiotics

No

Day 3

PUCAI >45 | PUCAI 35–45 | PUCAI <35

Screen for second-line therapy
surgical review
sigmoidoscopy (check for CMV)

Consider oral steroids
plan maintenance therapy

Day 5–11

PUCAI >65 | PUCAI 35–65 | PUCAI <35

Start second-line therapy
ciclosporin, tacrolimus or infliximab
or proceed to colectomy

Continue steroids with daily
review and re-enter algorithm
depending on PUCAI score

Day 7–14

PUCAI >65 | PUCAI 35–65 | PUCAI <35

Colectomy ← Consider continuing second-line therapy

AxR, plain abdominal X-ray; CMV, cytomegalovirus; FBC, full blood count; PUCAI, paediatric ulcerative colitis activity score; U&E, urea and electrolytes.

Algorithm 10.2 Managing severe colitis

- ○ Topical mesalazine (1–2 g/day) or steroids (5–20 mg) in liquid, foam or suppositories are effective therapy for mild to moderate left-sided colitis or isolated rectal disease. However, single therapy with topical mesalazine or steroids for distal disease is less effective than a combination of oral and topical therapy
- ○ Oral prednisone 1–2 mg/kg (up to 60 mg) daily is indicated if 5-ASA is ineffective. The full dose should be given for 2–4 weeks, until remission is attained, then weaned over 4–6 weeks. Long-term treatment with prednisone has significant adverse effects and has not been shown to be effective
- ○ Azathioprine 2–2.5 mg/kg/day or 6-mercaptopurine 1–1.5 mg/kg/day is used in steroid-dependent disease
- Acute illness and chronic symptoms should prompt review by a specialist centre. An assessment of disease severity and/or complications guides first-line treatment (see Algorithm 10.3). Third-line immune suppressants may be used if failure to respond or to wean from steroids, e.g. ciclosporin, tacrolimus, infliximab

Outcome

Acute severe colitis had a mortality rate of up to 30% before corticosteroid therapy. Up to 50% of acute severe colitis cases will require colectomy within 12 months.

Chronic colitis leads to a high risk of dysplasia, with risk of carcinoma. Screening is advised 10 years after diagnosis.

Inflammatory bowel disease specialist nurses

Key roles are:
- Patient/family support
- Information sharing and advice
- Transition to adult services, including sexual and reproductive health
- Medication advice
- Education issues

Patient education

A patient can form a very effective partnership with their healthcare professionals to allow improved management and prevention of complications from poor treatment compliance or unrecognised side-effects

UK Support organisations include:
- Crohn's in Childhood Research Association (CiCRA) www.cicra.org
- Colitis and Crohn's UK www.nacc.org.uk
- The Crohn's and Colitis Foundation of America (CCFA) www.ccfa.org
- Digestive Diseases Foundation CORE www.corecharity.org.uk

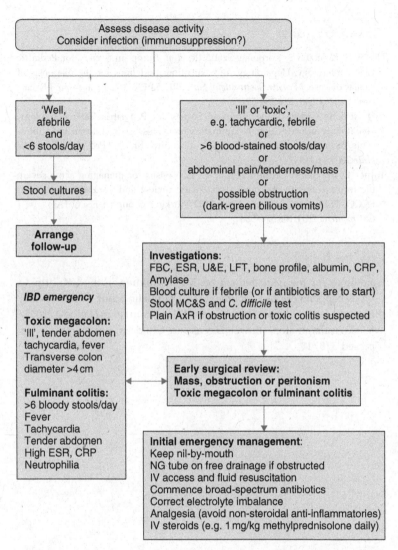

AxR, abdominal X-ray; CRP, C-reactive protein; ESR, erythrocyte sedimentation rate; FBC, full blood count; MC&S, microscopy, culture and sensitivity; NG, nasogastric; U&E, urea and electrolytes.

Algorithm 10.3 Management of an unwell child with inflammatory bowel disease

Further reading

Husby S, Koletzko S, Korponay-Szabó IR, *et al*. European Society for Pediatric Gastroenterology, Hepatology, and Nutrition guidelines for the diagnosis of coeliac disease. *J Pediatr Gastroenterol Nutr* 2012;54:136–160. Erratum in: *J Pediatr Gastroenterol Nutr* 2012;54:572

IBD Working Group of the European Society for Paediatric Gastroenterology, Hepatology and Nutrition. Inflammatory bowel disease in children and adolescents: recommendations for diagnosis – the Porto criteria. *J Pediatr Gastroenterol Nutr* 2005;41(1):1–7

Turner D, Travis SP, Griffiths AM, *et al*. Consensus for managing acute severe ulcerative colitis in children: a systematic review and joint statement from ECCO, ESPGHAN, and the Porto IBD Working Group of ESPGHAN. *Am J Gastroenterol* 2011;106:574–588

Key web links

Guidelines for the management of IBD in children in the UK: http://www.bspghan.org.uk/documents/IBDGuidelines.pdf

IBD diagnostic criteria: http://journals.lww.com/jpgn/Fulltext/2005/07000/Inflammatory_Bowel_Disease_in_Children_and.1.aspx – accessed 3/8/13

Gastrointestinal bleeding

The presence of blood in the vomitus or stool is never normal, and is alarming to families, but most cases have a benign cause. Causes vary by age and, in all groups, massive haemorrhage is rare, but challenging to manage.

Causes (see Table 11.1)

The vomitus or stool should be inspected as colorants may be mistaken for blood or altered blood. Iron therapy darkens stool and can be mistaken for maleana.

The colour of the blood in stool is indicative of the site of bleeding:
- Black: upper GI tract, e.g. varices
- Claret: midgut, e.g. Meckel's
- Red: lower bowel, e.g. fissure, polyp, colitis

Investigations (see Algorithm 11.1)

- FBC: anaemia or thrombocytopoenia
- Coagulation screen:
  - Prolonged PT suggests liver disease or vitamin K deficiency
  - Prolonged APTT suggests factor deficiency or other coagulopathy: seek Haematology advice
- Liver function tests
- Consider sepsis, especially infants
- Apt's test for maternal haemogloblin in neonates or breast-fed infants
- Meckel's scan: if abdominal pain and/or claret-coloured stool
- Endoscopy/colonoscopy: seek specialist advice

Practical Approach to Paediatric Gastroenterology, Hepatology and Nutrition, First Edition. Deirdre Kelly, Ronald Bremner, Jane Hartley, and Diana Flynn.
© 2014 John Wiley & Sons, Ltd. Published 2014 by John Wiley & Sons, Ltd.

Table 11.1 Causes of gastrointestinal bleeding

	Upper	Upper and lower	Lower
Infant	Swallowed maternal blood	Vitamin K deficiency (HDN)	Necrotising enterocolitis
			Anal fissure
		Haemangioma	Milk/soy allergy
		Intestinal duplication	Intussusception
			Bacterial gastroenteritis
			Polyp
			Meckel's
			Volvulus
Child/ adolescent	Swallowed blood	Coagulopathy	Bacterial gastroenteritis
		Tumour	Inflammatory bowel diseases
	Oesophagitis	Foreign body	
	Gastritis		Anal fissure
	Peptic ulcer (Figure 11.1)	Trauma (incl. abuse)	Haemorrhoids
		Angiodysplasia	Meckel's (Figure 11.2)
	Mallory–Weiss tear	Arteriovenous malformation	Volvulus
	Varices		Henoch–Schönlein purpura
	Caustic ingestion	Hereditary haemorrhagic telangiectasia	Polyp/polyposis
		Haemobilia	Heamolytic uraemic syndrome
			Lymphonodular hyperplasia?

HDN, haemolytic disease of the newborn.

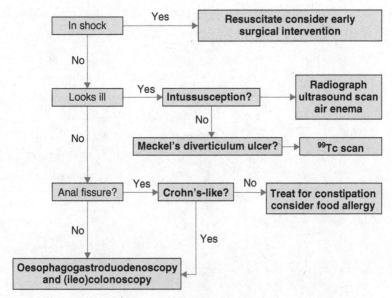

Algorithm 11.1 Investigation of lower gastrointestinal bleeding

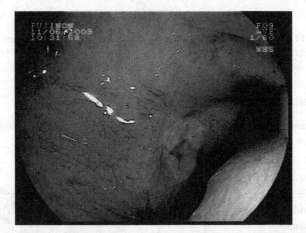

Figure 11.1 Endoscopic appearance of a pale ulcer in the duodenal cap with mild surrounding erythema, without evidence of recent bleeding and no visible vessel. This case presented with abdominal pain and malaena. There was associated *Helicobacter pylori* infection and antral gastritis.

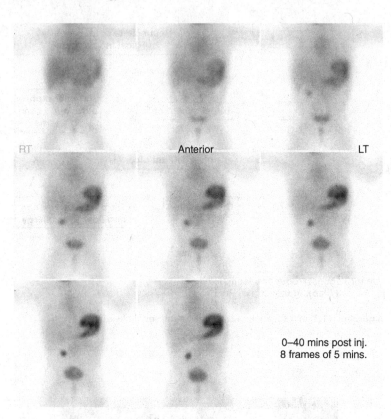

RT Anterior LT

0–40 mins post inj.
8 frames of 5 mins.

Figure 11.2 Gamma-emitting ^{99}Tc scan appearances of a Meckel's diverticulum, with uptake in the right iliac fossa, suggesting ectopic gastric mucosa. This infant presented with dark followed by bright red blood passed per rectum.

Management of upper GI bleeding

The management of upper GI bleeding including variceal bleeding is in Chapter 26.

Information: Polyposis

Presenting features
- Anaemia
- Lower GI bleeding
- Tenesmus
- Prolapse of rectum or polyp
- Intussusception or protein-losing enteropathy (rare)

Secondary screening of relatives with young-onset bowel cancer is required.

Juvenile polyps

- Clinical features: usually single or few (<5); usually in the left colon (Figure 11.3A)
- Histology: well differentiated cells lining dilated glands with inflammatory infiltrate
- Outcome: can recur, periodic colonoscopy if adenomatous

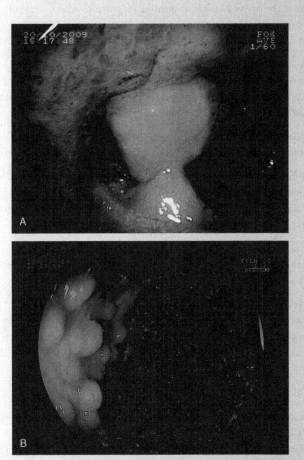

Figure 11.3 Endoscopic view of the left colon showing (A) a single large juvenile polyp and (B) multiple small polyps in a teenager with familial adenomatous polyposis.

(Continued)

Familial adenomatous polyposis coli and Gardener's syndrome
- Incidence: 1 in 50 000
- Most cases are found through family screening; *APC* gene mutation, some new mutations
- Gardener's syndrome: osteomas and soft tissue tumours
- Clinical features: hundreds of adenomas, unusually first seen in the left colon, with malignant transformation common in the third decade onwards (Figure 11.3B)
- Colectomy, usually with restorative ileal pouch procedure, is advised around the age of 20 years, depending on polyp numbers, size and severity of dysplasia
- Upper bowel polyps are more problematic to manage

PTEN–hamartoma–tumour syndromes
- Autosomal dominant; PTEN tumour suppressor gene associated
- Histology: hamartomatous polyps; not at very high risk of malignant transformation

Juvenile polyposis
- Clinical features: autosomal dominant; polyps in large and small bowel

Peutz–Jeghers syndrome
- Clinical features: lip and oral mucosal freckles; polyps, often in the jejunum and ileum, cause pain and risk of intussusception
- Malignancy risk: polyps, breast, ovary, Sertoli-derived tumours

Cowden syndrome
- Clinical features: colon and stomach polyps; hyperkeratotic papillomas of lips, tongue and nares; fibrocystic breast disease; thyroid adenoma

Bannayan–Riley–Ruvalcaba syndrome
- Clinical features: polyps of colon and tongue; macrocephaly; hypotonia; myopathy; developmental delay; arteriovenous malformations

Key web links

NICE Guideline for upper GI bleeding (2012): http://guidance.nice.org.uk/CG141

SIGN Guideline for upper and lower GI bleeding (2008): http://www.sign.ac.uk/guidelines/fulltext/105/index.html

Food-associated symptoms

Food stuffs induce symptoms by allergy (immune mediated) or intolerance (non-immune mechanism) which may be from malabsorption, such as in coeliac disease. In many cases, the mechanism of intolerance is not identifiable and is the result of a functional bowel disorder, not a pathological process. Such children may suffer from excessive investigation and/or an overly restricted diet, with consequent nutritional impairment.

Assessment (see Table 12.1)

Allergic responses are reproducible in onset, duration and clinical features. Triggers are proteins, sugars, chemicals and colorants. Maternal diet may cause allergy in a breast-fed infant. Delayed responses are more difficult to assess. Intolerances are often more unpredictable and variable.

Lactose (and other disaccharide) intolerance is a common secondary event after infection, with coeliac disease, food allergic enteropathy and inflammatory bowel disease. The duration is variable.

Important features from history

- Personal history of atopic disease: asthma, eczema or hayfever
- Family history of atopic disease or food allergy
- Details of foods that are avoided and the reasons why
- Specific questions:
  - Age of the child or young person when symptoms first started?
  - Speed of onset of symptoms following food contact?

Practical Approach to Paediatric Gastroenterology, Hepatology and Nutrition, First Edition.
Deirdre Kelly, Ronald Bremner, Jane Hartley, and Diana Flynn.
© 2014 John Wiley & Sons, Ltd. Published 2014 by John Wiley & Sons, Ltd.

Table 12.1 Assessment of food-induced illness

		Allergy		Intolerance
		IgE-mediated	Non-IgE mediated	
Symptoms	Rapid onset	+	–	±
	Onset after 6–48 hours	–	+	±
	Vomiting	+	–	±
	Diarrhoea	±	±	±
	Abdominal pain	±	+	+
	Gastro-oesophageal reflux	–	+	+
Signs	Urticaria/swelling/wheeze	+	±	–
	Other rashes/eczema	+	+	±
	Perianal irritation	–	±	±
	Blood in stools	–	±	–
Anaphylaxis		±	–	–
RAST/skin prick		±	–	–
Patch test		–	±	–
Food challenge		+	+	±
Intestinal biopsy		Normal	Variable	Normal

- ○ Duration of symptoms?
- ○ Severity of reaction
- ○ Frequency of occurrence
- ○ Setting of reaction, e.g. at school or home?
- ○ Reproducibility of symptoms on repeated exposure?
- ○ What food and how much exposure to it causes a reaction?
- ○ Who has raised the concern and suspects the food allergy?
- ○ What the suspected allergen is?
- Cultural and religious factors that affect the foods eaten
- Child or young person's feeding history: breast-fed or formula-fed, the age at which they were weaned – if the child is currently being breast-fed, consider the mother's diet
- Details of any previous treatment, including medication; any response to the elimination and re-introduction of foods

---

Information: Common food allergy triggers

- Cow's milk
- Soya bean (a legume)
- Egg
- Wheat
- Fish
- Shellfish
- Peanut
- Tree nuts, e.g. hazel, almond, pistachio

Investigations

The gold-standard test is the double-blind placebo-controlled cross-over food challenge, which is technically difficult and time-consuming. In practice, open food challenges are used.

- Allergy sensitisation tests:
  - ○ IgE-mediated allergy: RAST or skin prick testing for suspected triggers
  - ○ Non-IgE-mediated allergy: patch tests
  - ○ Results are difficult to interpret, because of false-negatives and non-specific sensitisation.
- Lactose, fructose or sucrose breath tests: small bowel or colonic intestinal bacteria ferment undigested sugars, producing hydrogen. A rise in hydrogen detected in exhaled breath is suggestive of a sugar malabsorption, especially when supported by a 48-hour symptom diary

- Evaluate further for non-allergic gastrointestinal disease if faltering growth and/or severe gastrointestinal symptoms have not responded to a single-allergen elimination diet; see Chapters 6, 9 and 10

Information: Cow's milk allergic colitis

- Presents with bright red blood streaks in stools
- Rarely hypoproteinaemia and oedema
- Typically endoscopy shows colonic lymphoid nodular hyperplasia
- Biopsies may show an eosinophilic inflammatory infiltrate
- Food protein-induced enteropathy syndrome (FPIES): a severe form can be mistaken for necrotising enterocolitis

---

Outcome

- Cow's milk and/or soya allergy will have resolved in 85% by age 2 years
- Food allergy is associated with atopic illness later in life

Coeliac disease

Coeliac disease is an immune-mediated systemic disorder in the genetically susceptible (HLA-DQ2 and DQ8 haplotypes). It is a sensitivity to gluten and related proteins, e.g. prolamins in oats, and characterised by a variable combination of gluten-dependent clinical manifestations, coeliac-specific antibodies and enteropathy.

Clinical features
Symptoms are very variable or absent.
- Persistent diarrhoea
- Faltering growth, idiopathic short stature
- Abdominal pain, vomiting, abdominal distension
- Constipation
- Dermatitis herpetiformis
- Dental enamel defects
- Osteoporosis/pathological fractures
- Delayed menarche
- Unexplained anaemia or iron-deficient anaemia unresponsive to treatment
- Recurrent aphthous stomatitis
- Unexplained liver disease
- Lassitude/weakness

- Incidence: 1 in 100–200, many cases undiagnosed, higher in associated conditions:
  - Type I diabetes (≥8%)
  - Selective IgA deficiency (1.7–7.7%)
  - Down's (5–12%), Williams' (8.2%) and Turner's (4.1–8.1%) syndromes
  - Autoimmune thyroiditis (~15%)
  - Autoimmune liver disease
  - Unexplained raised transaminases
- Relatives of coeliac patient:
  - First-degree relative (~10%)
  - HLA-matched sibling (~30–40%)
  - Monozygotic twin (~70%)
- Also consider: inflammatory arthritis, unexplained neurological problems (epilepsy, palsies, neuropathies, migraine)

Coeliac serology

- Antitissue transglutaminase: quantitative assay, cut-off limits vary between assays
- Antiendomysial antibody: qualitative immunofluorescence assay
- Anti-deamidated gliadin peptide antibody: less widely available
- Antigliadin antibody: unreliable

Investigation pathways are different for symptomatic and asymptomatic disease (see Algorithms 12.1 and 12.2).

Several endoscopic biopsies should be obtained from the first part of and the more distal duodenum (Figure 12.1).

Histology of duodenal biopsies (Figure 12.2) is graded using the Marsh criteria:

0. Normal appearance
1. Increased intraepithelial lymphocyte count
2. Lamina propria lymphocytic infiltration
3. Villous architecture abnormal

Management

- A life-long gluten-free diet. Gluten-free is defined as foods that contain 20 ppm or less. Supervision by a dietitian is necessary
- Accidental exposure is common
- Oats restricted initially, as often contaminated, but once in remission, gluten-free oats are re-introduced. Most are tolerant

Follow-up

- Assess symptoms, growth, adherence to gluten-free diet, dietary intake of calcium and iron

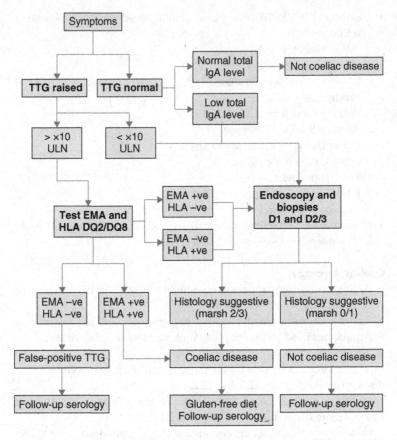

D1, first part of duodenum (bulb); D2/3, second or third part of duodenum; EMA, endomysial antibody test; HLA; human leukocyte antigen; TTG, tissue transglutaminase antibody titre; ULN, upper limit of normal (for TTG assay).

Algorithm 12.1 Investigation of suspected coeliac disease in symptomatic cases

- Check FBC, vitamin D level, and serology 6–12 months after starting gluten-free diet
- Advise pneumococcal vaccination (relative hyposplenism)
- Annual assessment and serology
- Introduce gluten-free oats after serology normalises
- Routine gluten challenge is not required

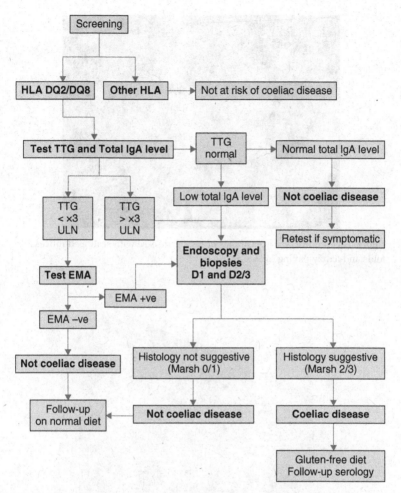

D1, first part of duodenum (bulb); D2/3, second or third part of duodenum; EMA, endomysial antibody test; HLA, human leukocyte antigen; TTG, tissue transglutaminase antibody titre; ULN, upper limit of normal (for TTG assay).

Algorithm 12.2 Investigation for asymptomatic coeliac disease and associated conditions

Outcome

- Compliance allows normal bone density and normal life expectancy
- Secondary lactose intolerance usually resolves
- Quality of life is improved
- Lifetime risk of small bowel lymphoma reduced

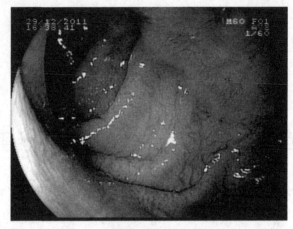

Figure 12.1 Endoscopic appearance of coeliac disease with scalloped mucosal folds and 'crazy paving' mucosal surface.

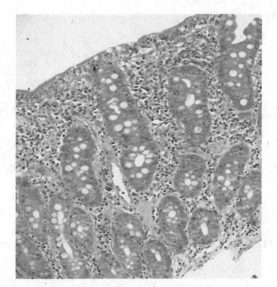

Figure 12.2 Histology of duodenal biopsies in coeliac disease, with intraepithelial lymphocytosis, a plasma-cell rich lamina propria chronic inflammatory infiltrate, crypt hyperplasia and flat mucosal surface (total villous atrophy). (Source: Courtesy of Dr M-A Brundler, Birmingham, UK.)

Information: Gluten challenge

- Indication: unclear diagnosis, on gluten-restriction
- Timing: avoid infancy and during pubertal growth
- Method:
  - 3 months daily gluten exposure (10–15 g/day) prior to serology testing is advised if asymptomatic with option to expedite blood testing when patient develops symptoms
  - Biopsy when serology becomes positive or symptoms are difficult to tolerate
  - A minimum duration of 4–6 weeks for those with symptoms during gluten challenge is recommended to maximise the likelihood of clear a diagnosis.
- Follow-up:
  - Follow-up for at least 2 years post challenge with serology at 6-monthly intervals if symptom free
  - Consider biopsy at 2 years even if asymptomatic
  - Late relapse occurs: advise gastroenterological assessment if symptoms suggestive of coeliac disease develop

---

Further reading

Husby S, Koletzko S, Korponay-Szabó IR, *et al*. European Society for Pediatric Gastroenterology, Hepatology, and Nutrition Guidelines for the Diagnosis of Coeliac Disease. *J Pediatr Gastroenterol Nutr* 2012;54:136–160

Key web links

BSPGHAN/CoeliacUK Guideline for diagnosis and management of coeliac disease in children: http://bspghan.org.uk/documents/Static/Coeliac%20Guidelines%202013.pdf
Celiac Disease Foundation (US): www.celiac.org
Coeliac UK: www.coeliac.org.uk

Abdominal mass

The normal infant may have a 1–2-cm smooth soft liver edge palpable in the right hypochondrium. Only occasionally is the spleen palpable in the normal child, and it tends to enlarge towards the left lower quadrant. The right kidney may be ballotable in a slim older child. Bowel loops are often palpable in the iliac fossae or suprapubic areas.

Routine ultrasound scanning may show an abdominal mass antenatally. Any mass should be investigated urgently.

Important features from history and examination

- Onset, variability and progression
- Weight loss
- Fever
- Evaluate for cardiac, kidney or liver disease
- Menstrual history, vaginal discharge and sexual activity
- Bleeding, bruising or pallor suggest haematological malignancy or coagulopathy
- Family history: haemaglobinopathy, metabolic diseases, renal cystic disease

Differential diagnosis and investigations

Distension without mass
- Malabsorption: see Chapter 6
- Ascites: see Chapter 25
- Bowel obstruction: see Chapter 4

Practical Approach to Paediatric Gastroenterology, Hepatology and Nutrition, First Edition.
Deirdre Kelly, Ronald Bremner, Jane Hartley, and Diana Flynn.
© 2014 John Wiley & Sons, Ltd. Published 2014 by John Wiley & Sons, Ltd.

- Constipation with impaction: see Chapter 15
- Aerophagia: Plain radiograph, early morning girth
- Perforation: Abdominal, erect chest or decubitus radiograph

Right upper quadrant
- Hepatomegaly: see Chapters 20 and 23
- Hepatoblastoma: serum alpha-fetoprotein
- Choledochal cyst: ultrasound or CT
- Gall bladder: ultrasound (consider Kawasaki's disease)

Right lower quadrant
- Intussusception: ultrasound, air/barium enema
- Appendiceal inflammatory mass: ultrasound or CT
- Crohn's disease: ultrasound, MRI enterography
- Meckel's diverticulum: ^{99}Tc scan, ultrasound or CT

Left upper quadrant
- Splenomegaly: see Chapters 20 and 23
- Pancreatic pseudocyst: serum amylase/lipase, ultrasound or CT

Renal masses
- Hydronephrosis: U&E, creatinine, ultrasound
- Wilm's tumour: ultrasound or CT
- Neuroblastoma: urine catecholamines (VMA, HVA, dopamine)
- Polycystic kidney disease: U&E, creatinine, ultrasound
- Renal vein thrombosis: ultrasound with Doppler studies

Subrapubic
- Faecal mass: none or plain radiograph
- Urinary retention: ultrasound, micturating cytourethrogram (MCUG)
- Hydro- or haemato-colpos: ultrasound or CT
- Ovarian cyst: ultrasound or CT

Any site
- Intestinal duplication cyst: ultrasound or CT
- Omental or mesenteric cyst: ultrasound or CT
- Teratoma   β-chorionic gonadotrophin, ultrasound or CT
- Lymphoma   FBC, LDH, uric acid; ultrasound or CT

> **Red flags: Concerning abdominal distension**
>
> - Neonatal abdominal distension may be the first sign of necrotising enterocolitis
> - Malignant abdominal masses are most often Wilms' tumour, neuroblastoma or lymphoma

Management

- Early involvement of paediatric surgeons and oncologist
- Specific management should be directed at managing the underlying causative process or disease

Further reading

NICE Guidelines on Cancer Services for Children and Young People: http://guidance.nice.org.uk/CSGCYP

Guidelines for managing necrotising entercolitis in premature infants: Cincinnati Children's Hospital (2010) http://www.guideline.gov/content.aspx?id=24815

Key web links

Family support for necrotising entercolitis in premature infants: http://kidshealth.org/parent/medical/digestive/nec.html

Support for children with cancer: http://www.macmillan.org.uk/Cancerinformation/Cancertypes/Childrenscancers/Childrenscancers.aspx

The infant with constipation

Stool frequency in infancy is very variable, and stools are often softer and passed more frequently by exclusively breast-fed children. Functional constipation is common in infants, usually a few weeks after birth and often following changes in diet or reduced fluid intake. Onset during weaning is common. Up to half of children with constipation develop it in the first year of life. Passage of a hard or large stool can cause an anal fissure, and then stool withholding behaviour to avoid the pain of passing a stool. This is can be inaccurately interpreted by carers as straining to pass stool.

Organic causes

- Anal fissure
- Anorectal anomalies: fistula or anterior anus
- Hirschsprung's disease: delayed passage of meconium, abdominal distension
- Sacral agenesis: patulous anus
- Hypothyroidism: infrequent stools, poor feeding, poor postnatal linear growth
- Cystic fibrosis: pale stools, oily stools, poor weight gain, respiratory symptoms
- Cow's milk protein intolerance/allergy: associated reflux, eczema, family history of atopy
- Coeliac disease: onset after introduction of weaning, associated faltering growth, abdominal distension, muscle wasting, iron-deficiency anaemia (see Chapter 12)
- Spinal dysraphism

Practical Approach to Paediatric Gastroenterology, Hepatology and Nutrition, First Edition.
Deirdre Kelly, Ronald Bremner, Jane Hartley, and Diana Flynn.
© 2014 John Wiley & Sons, Ltd. Published 2014 by John Wiley & Sons, Ltd.

Examination and investigations

- Assess stool character:
  - ○ Ribbon stools suggest Hirschsprung's disease
  - ○ Pale or oily stools suggest fat malabsorption (steatorrhoea)
  - ○ Red blood streaks suggest fissure, enterocolitis or allergic colitis
- Abdominal radiographs are rarely required, unless there is abdominal distension or suspected enterocolitis
- Screening blood tests: FBC, thyroid function, coeliac serology (if on gluten)
- In selected cases:
  - ○ Sweat test or cystic fibrosis genetic tests
  - ○ Rectal suction or strip biopsy for ganglion cells

Management

Suspected Hirschsprung's

- Nil-by-mouth, nasogastric drainage and intravenous fluids if obstructed
- Broad-spectrum IV antibiotics for enterocolitis
- Plain abdominal radiograph
- Seek urgent surgical advice: obstruction usually requires stoma formation
- Definitive surgery resects or bypasses the affected segments (Duhamel or Swenson procedure), with newer techniques using a transanal approach

Functional constipation

- Ensure adequate fluid intake
- Consider a trial of cow's milk free diet
- Osmotic laxative to soften stools, e.g. lactulose 5–10 mL twice daily
- Low-dose stimulant laxatives, e.g. senna syrup 2.5–5 mL once daily

Diet

Cow's milk protein intolerance or allergy can present with constipation, but it is not usually necessary to restrict cow's milk intake in an infant with constipation. If dietary restriction is required, the new diet should be checked to ensure nutritional adequacy, ideally by a paediatric dietitian or nutritional specialist.

Outcome

Functional constipation often responds well to therapy, although these infants are more likely to develop functional bowel disease in childhood.

Long-term dependence on laxative therapy and/or failure to achieve continence in slow-transit constipation can be managed by surgery, e.g. the antegrade colonic enema procedure. Criteria for case selection are not well established.

Hirschsprung's disease outcome is dependent on the length of bowel involved. Children with long-segment disease or total aganglionosis often have long-term intestinal failure (see Chapter 44).

Red flags: When to refer for constipation

- Poor unresponsive to initial therapy
- Abdominal distension
- Dilated bowel loops on plain radiography
- Suspected neuropathic bowel or pseudo-obstruction

Information: Hirschsprung's disease

This is a congenital aganglionosis of the Auerbach plexus and Meissner plexus of a variable length of the bowel, 70% have short segment disease, i.e. distal to the descending colon.

Presenting features
- Neonatal-onset constipation, often with features of bowel obstruction
- Delayed passage of meconium (>48 hours) in a term infant
- Enterocolitis
- Severe constipation with onset in the neonatal period and that is unresponsive to standard therapy, e.g. requiring suppositories or enemas

Examination findings
- Tympanic abdominal distension, with visible or palpable bowel loops
- Faltering growth
- An empty small rectum on per-rectal examination, with a gush of liquid stool on withdrawal of the digit. (NB: This can cause clinical decompensation in obstruction or enterocolitis, and must be performed only by an experienced practitioner)

(Continued)

Incidence
- 1 in 4500–5000 live births
- M:F 4:1

Genetics
- Multiple genes have been implicated: *RET*, endothelin B receptor, *GDNF*, endothelin-3
- 5–15% of children with trisomy 21 have Hirschsprung's disease
- Associated with Waardenburg syndrome

Investigations
- Diagnosis confirmed by absent ganglion cells in the rectal submucosa, obtained by suction biopsy 2–2.5 cm above the dentate line or a wedge resection biopsy
- Staining for acetylcholinesterase can identify hypertrophic extrinsic nerve trunks
- Skip lesions occur, especially in long-segment disease.

Further reading

Gordon M, Naidoo K, Akobeng AK, Thomas AG. Osmotic and stimulant laxatives for the management of childhood constipation. *Cochrane Database Syst Rev* 2012;Issue 7:CD009118

Kim AC, Langer JC, Pastor AC, *et al*. Endorectal pull-through for Hirschsprung's disease-a multicenter, long-term comparison of results: transanal vs transabdominal approach. *J Pediatr Surg* 2010;45:1213–1220

Key web links

Clinical guidelines: NICE CG99 Constipation in children and young people: http://www.nice.org.uk/cg99

NASPGHAN Clinical Practice Guideline: http://www.naspghan.org/user-assets/Documents/pdf/PositionPapers/constipation.guideline.2006.pdf

http://onlinelibrary.wiley.com/doi/10.1002/14651858.CD009118.pub2/full

Family support:

Education and resources for improving childhood continence: http://www.eric.org.uk

Information, education, support and advocacy for families, children, teens and adults who are living with the challenges of congenital anorectal, colorectal or urogenital disorders: http://www.pullthrunetwork.org

Hirshprung's disease and motility disorders support: http://www.hirschsprungs.info

The child with constipation

Difficulty passing stool, the passage of hard stool or the infrequent passage of stool is a common complaint, affecting up to 30% of children. It is a common reason for referral, accounting for up to 5% of all paediatric outpatient visits. Constipation may become chronic, leading to stool impaction and incomplete rectal emptying. It is a functional disorder, but may be caused by organic disease, including cystic fibrosis and perianal Crohn's disease. Immobility and/or neurological disorders are commonly associated with constipation.

Presenting symptoms

Onset is often around the time of toilet training, commencing nursery/ school or during periods of upset of routine (moving house, admission to hospital, family disruption).
- Stool character:
  - Passage of three or fewer stools per week
  - Small hard stools ('rabbit droppings')
  - Large stools ('toilet blockers')
  - Faecal soiling, often without sensation
  - Overflow diarrhoea
- Behaviours:
  - Retentive posturing: back arching, tiptoes, legs crossed, squatting
  - Straining or distress during defaecation or attempting to withhold stool
  - Hiding when passing a stool or withholding
  - Reduced appetite and/or misery, improved following passage of a stool

Practical Approach to Paediatric Gastroenterology, Hepatology and Nutrition, First Edition.
Deirdre Kelly, Ronald Bremner, Jane Hartley, and Diana Flynn.
© 2014 John Wiley & Sons, Ltd. Published 2014 by John Wiley & Sons, Ltd.

- ○ Toilet phobia
- ○ Nocturnal enuresis or daytime wetting
- Pain:
  - ○ Central or lower abdominal pain, often prior or after passage of stool
  - ○ Anal pain (see Chapter 16)
- Abdominal distension, relieved by defaecation
- Bright red blood per rectum, or on wiping, suggests fissure or minor prolapse
- Encopresis (passage of stool in abnormal places) – not always due to constipation
- Soiling (faecal incontinence) – not always due to constipation

Physical findings

- Faltering growth: consider organic disease or abuse (harm or neglect)
- Abdominal inspection: distension suggests significant colonic stool loading, aerophagia or obstruction
- Abdominal palpation: a subrapubic mass suggests sigmoid loading and/or impaction
- Legs: abnormal gait or deep tendon reflexes suggest a neurological cause
- Sacral/gluteal region:
  - ○ Abnormal muscle bulk or sacral appearance suggests sacral agenesis
  - ○ Midline naevus, pit/sinus or scoliosis suggests spinal anomaly
- Perianal inspection:
  - ○ Anal position, anal 'wink' (reflex contraction and transient relaxation)
  - ○ Patulous anus suggests lower motor neurone damage
  - ○ Perianal erythema suggests streptococcal skin infection
  - ○ Perianal fistulae suggest Crohn's disease
  - ○ Superficial anal fissures suggest passage of hard and/or large stools
- Digital per rectum examination is rarely indicated, and if required should be undertaken by a professional experienced in the assessment of anorectal anomalies or Hirschsprung's disease

Assessment

- Toileting behaviour, location, duration, frequency for urination and defaecation

- Stool form, e.g. Bristol stool form chart
- Fluid intake, diet and eating habits
- Sensation: 'the call to stool'
- Inquire about toilet refusal or phobia
- Be aware of signs of child abuse
- Inpatient admission may help define which factors are important, offer respite to families and allow thorough disimpaction before initiating a maintenance strategy

Investigations

- Blood tests:
  - Blood count: anaemia secondary to occult GI blood loss
  - Antitissue transglutaminase and/or endomysial antibodies: coeliac disease
  - Thyroid function: hypothyroidism
  - Bone biochemistry: hypoparathyroidism
  - (Lead levels: lead poisoning)
  - (Creatine kinase: myopathy)
- Imaging:
  - Abdominal radiography is rarely required, but may assess the degree of stool loading of rectum and colon when managing faecal impaction
  - Transit marker studies are reserved for selected cases with poor response to therapy, or if a motility disorder is suspected
  - Spinal magnetic resonance scan: assesses spinal cord anatomy if there is a scoliosis, sacral anomaly or spinal bifida occulta
- Full thickness rectal mucosal biopsy for suspected Hirschsprung's disease
- Colonic transit marker studies:
  - Normal oro-anal transit time is up to 48 hours
  - Radio-opaque markers of different shapes are ingested over a period of 3 days and then plain radiographs repeated from day 4 to day 7
  - Retained markers in the colon or part of the colon can suggest a diffuse or segmental dysmotility
- Anorectal and colonic manometry: a research tool in paediatrics, reserved for the assessment of motility disorders
- Defaecating proctography: a real-time radiographic assessment of anorectal and pelvic muscle function used in adults. Radiation doses and acceptance limit its use in children

---

Red flags: When to be concerned

- Delayed passage of meconium (after 48 hours of age in a term infant)
- Onset in the neonatal period
- Abnormal neurology
- 'Ribbon' stools: suggests Hirschsprung's disease
- Steatorrhoea: suggests malabsorption, e.g. cystic fibrosis
- Disclosure/history or signs of child abuse
- Gross abdominal distension or with vomiting: suggests obstruction
- Anaemia
- Faltering growth

Management

Information and explanation

A central part of management is to demystify the process of defaecation and toileting behaviour, and to understand the psychosocial context. Parents' and child's expectations need to be understood and met to be able to agree a management strategy that can be maintained over a long time period. Re-iteration during follow-up is often required.

Dietary management

- Oral fluid intake should be adequate, but not excessive
- Dietary fibre manipulation is rarely useful, and increasing dietary insoluble fibre, e.g. bran, may worsen symptoms by increasing stool bulk without softening, and causing flatulence
- There is no evidence of benefit from probiotics

Toileting

A routine of sitting on the toilet after meals in the morning and evening encourages regular bowel movements, which is central to managing functional constipation. Stool withholding increases the likelihood of colonic loading, therefore impaction and overflow soiling. Thus, withholding should be addressed by encouraging toiling when the 'call to stool' is recognised. This routine is established using positive reinforcement of behaviours, appropriate to developmental stage, in a non-confrontational manner. Colonic motility is promoted by physical activity.

Biofeedback training with anorectal manometry is rarely used in children.

Medical management
Laxative medications are used to support behavioural modifications.

Disimpation
This is for colonic loading that prevents effective rectal emptying.

Rectally administered treatments can cause distress. The negative association of rectally administered treatment and the sensations of stool passage can make progress towards normal toileting behaviour more difficult. Disimpaction can usually be achieved using oral macrogols, e.g. Movicol, KleenPrep, alone or together with a stimulant. Doses should be individualised, and if standard doses are insufficient, then refer for specialist review.

Maintenance treatment
Once stooling is established, laxative support can be withdrawn slowly, usually over a period of months, with the aim of using the minimum required dose to support rectal emptying. Relapse is common, requiring dose escalation. Passage of very soft stools may represent either overflow secondary to impaction or laxative effect.

Outcome

Follow-up
A multidisciplinary support network for the family and patient and regular reassessment are important components of successful management of chronic constipation. Soiling frequency is often a poor marker of success, and focus should be on the passage of stool in the toilet.

Complications
- Acquired megarectum: with prolonged rectal loading, there is compensatory rectal dilatation, reducing rectal muscle tone and further impairing emptying. This process is usually reversible, but may take many months
- Psychosocial issues: continence issues often affect confidence and social interactions within families and beyond. Peer relationships can be compromised and affected children subject to bullying
- Intractable constipation: if medical and behavioural management fails, then assessment of colonic motility and psychological interventions should be considered as part of an assessment by a specialist team. Rarely, in severe cases unresponsive to conventional treatment, quality of life can be improved with surgical procedures, e.g. antegrade colonic enema

---

Information: Oral laxatives

These are suggested initial doses. Higher doses are often required in chronic constipation with colonic loading and/or megarectum.

- Osmotic laxatives:
  - ○ Lactulose: 1–2 mL/kg, in two or three divided doses daily
  - ○ Polyethylene glycol 3350 plus electrolytes (Movicol Paediatric Plain, KleenPrep) 2–4 sachets daily with water or juice
- Stimulant laxatives:
  - ○ Senna (syrup, granules or tablets) 7.5–30 mg at night
  - ○ Docusate sodium 12.5–25 mg twice daily
  - ○ Bisacodyl 5–10 mg at night
  - ○ Sodium picosulphate 2.5–10 mg at night

Information: Distal intestinal obstruction syndrome in cystic fibrosis (CF)

Viscous secretions obstruct the distal ileum in 10–20% of patients with CF.

Presenting features
- Progressive recurrent abdominal pain, bloating, nausea, anorexia, abdominal distension, fatty stools and constipation
- Partial or complete small bowel obstruction, with a tender mass in the right iliac fossa

Investigations
- Plain abdominal radiograph: faecal loading in right iliac fossa, empty colon, dilated small bowel

Management
- Small bowel lavage: Gastrograffin, macrogol (KleenPrep, Movicol) or N-acetylcysteine
- Review pancreatic enzyme replacement doses
- Surgery may be required in unresponsive cases

Differential diagnosis
- Intussussception or inflammatory mass: ultrasound and/or CT scan, colonoscopy
- Fibrosing colonopathy
- Pancreatitis

Outcome
- 50% recurrence

Key web links

Clinical practice guideline: www.nice.org.uk/guidance/CG99
Patient/parent support: www.eric.org.uk/www.ibsnetwork.org
Education and resources for improving childhood continence:
  http://www.eric.org.uk

Perianal pain

Specific questions may be required to elicit this symptom, and there may be no clue from the history in a pre-school child. A high index of suspicion and careful clinical examination can help identify the common causes of pain and constipation (Table 16.1). Perianal abscess should alert to the possibility of Crohn's disease and early surgical referral.

Practical Approach to Paediatric Gastroenterology, Hepatology and Nutrition, First Edition.
Deirdre Kelly, Ronald Bremner, Jane Hartley, and Diana Flynn.
© 2014 John Wiley & Sons, Ltd. Published 2014 by John Wiley & Sons, Ltd.

Table 16.1 Causes, investigation and treatment of perianal pain

Cause	Typical features	Investigation	Treatment	Outcome
Anal fissure and/or haemorrhoids	Red blood in stool, sharp perianal pain with stooling, pain on wiping	Consider pelvis MRI for Crohn's disease and/or fistula	Laxatives: topical 0.05–0.1% glyceryl trinitrate ointment prn	Often recurrent
Threadworms	Nocturnal itch	Sticky tape test	Mebendazole 100 mg two doses, 2 weeks apart	Re-infestation common
Streptococcal skin infection	Bright red shiny perianal skin	Skin swab for culture	Penicillin V 250–500 mg qds for 10–14 days Clarithromycin 125–250 mg bd for 10–14 days	Antibiotic resistance common
Proctlagia fugax	Sudden severe anal or rectal pain, lasting seconds or minutes	None	Inhaled salbutamol 400–800 µg at pain onset	Episodic or in clusters Associated with irritable bowel syndrome

Hepatology

Liver disease in childhood is rare but important. Many children need specialist treatment so it is best to discuss and refer cases to a paediatric hepatology specialist, particularly to decide when a liver transplant is required. This section provides an overview of liver disease. We have highlighted the common conditions and alert the reader to common pitfalls or essential information for immediate management.

Practical Approach to Paediatric Gastroenterology, Hepatology and Nutrition, First Edition.
Deirdre Kelly, Ronald Bremner, Jane Hartley, and Diana Flynn.
© 2014 John Wiley & Sons, Ltd. Published 2014 by John Wiley & Sons, Ltd.

The infant with jaundice

Jaundice is common in newborn infants. Physiological jaundice occurs from day 3 after birth and resolves by 2 weeks of age. Benign unconjugated hyperbilirubinaemia may persist beyond this time due to the influence of breast milk oestrogens, but any infant who has persistent jaundice (>2 weeks) requires investigation.

Red flags: When to be concerned about jaundice

- Any infant who has persistent jaundice after 2 weeks should have a split bilirubin test to distinguish between unconjugated and conjugated jaundice
- Conjugated hyperbilirubinaemia indicates liver disease requiring referral to a liver specialist centre for urgent investigation.

Important features from history

- Family history of jaundice, neonatal deaths or miscarriages
- Low or normal birth weight, failure to thrive or weight loss
- Poor feeding and irritability
- Hypoglycaemic episodes
- Vitamin K deficiency with bleeding

Examination

- Babies with significant liver disease may have a normal birth weight and normal physical examination
- Dysmorphic features, arthrogryposis, cutaneous haemangioma

Practical Approach to Paediatric Gastroenterology, Hepatology and Nutrition, First Edition.
Deirdre Kelly, Ronald Bremner, Jane Hartley, and Diana Flynn.
© 2014 John Wiley & Sons, Ltd. Published 2014 by John Wiley & Sons, Ltd.

- Cardiac murmur
- Enlarged spleen: always an abnormal sign
- Ascites

Investigations (Algorithm 17.1 and Algorithm 17.2)

The differential diagnosis and investigations for causes of unconjugated jaundice are shown in Table 17.1 and causes of conjugated jaundice are shown in Table 17.2.

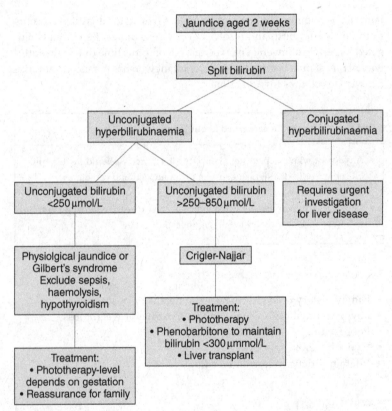

Algorithm 17.1 Investigating a 2-week-old infant with jaundice

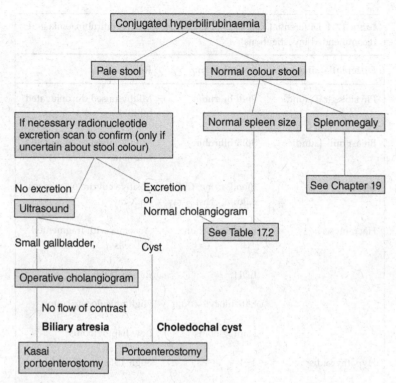

Algorithm 17.2 Investigating conjugated hyperbilirubinaemia at 2 weeks of age

Table 17.1 Differential diagnosis of unconjugated hyperbilirubinaemia and recommended investigations

Differential diagnosis	Investigation	Results
Physiological jaundice	Split bilirubin	Mildly raised unconjugated bilirubin
Breast milk jaundice	Split bilirubin	Mildly raised unconjugated bilirubin
Sepsis	Blood, urine, CSF culture, chest X-ray	Positive culture or changes on X-ray
Haemolysis	Full blood count	Anaemia with fragmented red cells
	LDH	Raised LDH
	Reticulocyte count	High reticulocyte count
	Haptoglobins	Low haptoglobins
Hypothyroidism	TFTs	High TSH
		Low T4
Pyloric stenosis	Ultrasound scan	Thickening of the gastric pylorus muscle. Excessive gastric peristalsis
Gilbert's syndrome	Split bilirubin	Mild unconjugated hyperbilirubinaemia
Crigler–Najjar I and II	Split bilirubin	Significantly raised unconjugated hyperbilirubinaemia requiring treatment (see Algorithm 17.1)

CSF, cerebrospinal fluid; LDH, lactate dehydrogenase; TFT, thyroid function test; TSH, thyroid stimulating hormone.

Table 17.2 Differential diagnosis of conjugated hyperbilirubinaemia when biliary atresia has been excluded, and recommended investigations and treatment

Differential diagnosis	Investigation	Results	Specific treatment
Alpha-1-antitrypsin deficiency	Level and protein phenotype	Low alpha-1-antitrypsin level	General management of cholestasis (see below)
		PiZZ phenotype	
Hypothyroidism	TFTs	Raised TSH	Thyroxine replacement
		Low T4	
Hypopituitarism	TFT, cortisol, glucose	Low TSH, cortisol Hypoglycaemia	Replace hormone deficiency
Galactosaemia	Urine reducing substances	Positive reducing substances	Galactose-free diet
	Plasma Gal-1-Put	Absent or reduced Gal-1-Put detected	
Tyrosinaemia	Urine succinyl acetone	High succinyl acetone	NTBC (nitisinone), low tyrosine diet
	DNA	Mutations in *FAH*	

(Continued)

Table 17.2 (*Continued*)

Differential diagnosis	Investigation	Results	Specific treatment
Alagille syndrome	Echocardiography	Peripheral pulmonary stenosis, Butterfly-shaped thoracic vertebrae	Management of cholestasis (see below)
	Thoracic vertebrae X-ray		
	Slit-lamp examination	Posterior embryotoxon	
	DNA	*JAG1* or *NOTCH2* mutations	
Congenital infection	Serology urine and blood, PCR-CMV, toxoplasma,	Positive testing	Ganciclovir may be beneficial for congenital CMV
Progressive familial intrahepatic cholestasis 1 and 2	GGT	Low GGT cholestasis	Management of cholestasis (see below)
	Liver biopsy	Specific findings on histology	
	DNA	Mutation in *ATP8B1* or *ABCB11*	
Arthrogryposis, renal dysfunction cholestasis (ARC) syndrome	GGT	Low GGT cholestasis	Management of cholestasis (see below)
	DNA	Mutation in *VPS33B* or *VIPAR*	

Condition	Investigation	Result	Management
Storage disease, e.g. Neimann Pick C	Liver biopsy / Bone marrow biopsy / Filipin staining / DNA	Storage cells on bone marrow and liver biopsy (can be difficult to see in young children) / Positive Filipin staining of fibroblasts / Mutation in NPC1 and 2	Management of cholestasis (see below)
Bile salt synthesis disorders	Urinary bile salts (not accurate if on ursodeoxycholic acid) / DNA	Abnormal peaks on urine mass spectroscopy / Mutation in AKR1D1	Cholic acid
Citrin deficiency	Plasma and urine amino acids / DNA	Increased plasma and urine citrulline and arginine / Mutation in SLC25A13	Supportive with management of cholestasis
Peroxisomal disorders	Plasma very long chain fatty acids / DNA	High levels of very long chain fatty acids / Mutation in PEX genes	Palliation
Intestinal failure-associated liver disease	Liver biopsy	Specific findings on liver biopsy	Ursodeoxycholic acid / Encourage enteral diet / Prompt treatment of sepsis

CMV, cytomegalovirus; GGT, gamma-glutamyl transpeptidase; PCR, polymerase chain reaction; TFT, thyroid function test; TSH, thyroid stimulating hormone.

Information: Biliary atresia

Any infant with conjugated hyperbilirubinaemia should be investigated for biliary atresia at a specialist liver unit. Biliary atresia is a progressive obliterative cholangiopathy which prevents bile flow into the intestine. The aetiology is unclear but may be a complex interaction between genetic predisposition, immunological potential and infective agents. In up to 20% of cases there is polysplenia, preduodenal portal vein and cardiac defects.

Clinical signs include failure to thrive, pale stools, dark urine (Figure 17.1). On ultrasound there may be an absent or small gallbladder (Figure 17.2).

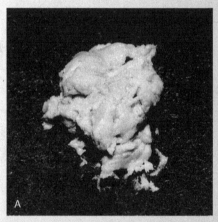

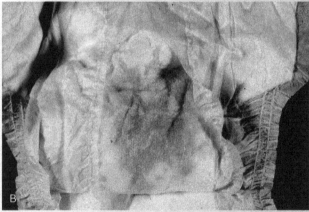

Figure 17.1 (A,B) Pale stool and dark urine. In babies with an obstruction to bile flow such as biliary atresia the urine is dark and the stools pale. In biliary atresia the stools may become gradually paler until white by 6 weeks of age.

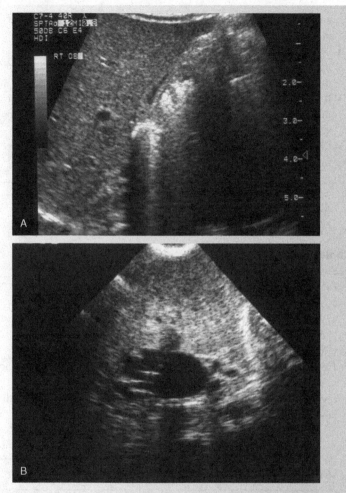

Figure 17.2 Ultrasound scan images showing (A) an absent gallbladder after a 4-hour fast in biliary atresia and (B) an echo-lucent round lesion in choledochal cyst.

Management

- The Kasai portoenterostomy is a palliative surgical procedure to re-establish flow of bile and is more successful when carried out early (preferably before 60 days). Hence, it is important to identify infants with biliary atresia early
- A successful Kasai is achieved in approximately 60% of cases and is defined as a normal bilirubin 6 months after the procedure. Infants with

(Continued)

an unsuccessful operation require liver transplantation in the first year of life
- 90% of children with a successful Kasai develop cirrhosis and portal hypertension and require long-term follow-up to manage chronic liver disease and the need for liver transplantation
- If there is pyrexia, irritability, abdominal pain or pale stools post Kasai, then treat for cholangitis with 10–14 days of IV antibiotics, e.g. Tazocin 90 mg/kg/dose tds
- Cholangitis is the main cause of liver decompensation and transplantation.

Management

Cholestasis
- Ensure optimum nutrition to address fat malabsorption
- Fat-soluble vitamins: recommended vitamin doses in infancy:
  - Vitamin A 5000 units once daily
  - Vitamin E 50 mg once daily
  - Alpha calcidol 100 ng/kg once daily
  - Vitamin K 1 mg daily
- Treat pruritis which causes sleep loss and interference with daily activities (see Chapter 24)
- Liver transplant for decompensated liver disease, failure to thrive despite intensive nutritional support or intractable pruritis

---

Information: Low GGT cholestasis

In most cases of cholestasis the GGT is high. Low GGT cholestasis suggests bile salt transport defects: progressive familial intrahepatic cholestasis (PFIC) 1 and 2 (mutations in *ATP8B7* and *ABCB11*, respectively), bile salt synthesis disorder (*AKR1D1*) or ARC (*VPS33B* or *VIPAR*) syndrome. These disorders present with jaundice, progressive liver disease, pruritis or fat-soluble vitamin deficiency.

Clinical features
- PFIC1: diarrhoea (which may only become evident following transplantation) and deafness
- ARC syndrome: arthrogryposis, renal deficiency and poor platelet function which precludes liver biopsy

Management
- Nutritional support
- Management of cholestasis
- Supplementation of bile salts (cholic acid) in bile salt synthesis defects

Outcome
- PFIC1 and 2: transplant is usually required during childhood
- ARC syndrome: death occurs in the first year of life
- Bile salt transport defects: liver disease stabilises with cholic acid supplementation and transplantation may not be required

---

Information: Alagille syndrome

This autosomal dominant disease (mutations in *JAG1* or *NOTCH2*) has a diverse phenotypic presentation.

Clinical features
- Cholestasis
- Dysmorphism with broad forehead
- Hypertelorism and pointed chin
- Skeletal anomalies including butterfly vertebrae
- Posterior embryotoxon of the eyes
- Cardiac disease with peripheral pulmonary stenosis
- Failure to thrive
- Fat malabsorption, fat-soluble vitamin deficiency
- Pruritis

Management
- Nutritional support
- Liver transplantation is rarely required

Information: Alpha-1-antitrypsin deficiency (A1AT deficiency)

This is the most common autosomal recessive inherited liver disease in Caucasians.
   The protein phenotype PiZZ is associated with liver disease.

Clinical features
- Cholestasis in the neonate
- Portal hypertension or abnormal liver function tests in childhood

(Continued)

Management
- Management of cholestasis

Outcome
- Cholestasis resolves in most
- Long-term follow-up is necessary to identify progressive liver disease, which may require treatment for portal hypertension and liver transplantation

Nutrition

Nutrition is an essential part of managing children with liver disease and improves the outcome. Cholestasis reduces the absorption of long-chain triglycerides (LCTs) and therefore a formula with a higher content of medium-chain triglycerides (MCTs) is necessary (see Table 17.3). A feeding history may indicate a child is having a good intake of feed but the high energy requirements of liver disease combined with the lack of LCT absorption means the child may not thrive.

Weight for age is not a reliable indicator of nutritional progress because organomegaly, ascites and oedema can mask weight loss. Serial mid-arm circumference and triceps skinfold estimate muscle bulk and fat stores, and decline before changes in weight or height are apparent as they are not influenced by oedema.

Nutritional requirements for infants with cholestatic liver disease are:
- Increase energy 100–150 kcal/kg/day
- 10% energy from protein or 3–6 g protein/kg/day
- 30–50% energy from fat, 30–70% fat as MCT

Table 17.3 Products used in paediatric liver disease (per 100 mls)

Feed	Kcals	Protein (g)	Fat (% MCT)	Na (mmol)	EFA's $\Omega 6: \Omega 3$
Pregestimil	68	1.9	55%	1.3	16.8:1
Peptijunior	67	1.8	50%	0.9	5.4:1
Infatrini Peptisorb	100	2.6	50%	1.4	4.18:1
Heparon Junior	86.4	2	50%	0.56	
MCT Pepdite	68	2	75%	1.5	6.9:1
Modular feed	70–200	Flexible	0–100%	0–1.5 mmol/kg	None

EFAs, essential fatty acids.

If on normal infant formula

If the infant has a bilirubin level of greater than 70 μmol/L with poor growth and/or over feeding on normal formula, change to an MCT-containing feed until cholestasis resolves. If poor weight gain persists, concentrate formula and add calories from carbohydrate polymers and fat emulsions.

If breast-feeding

Continue breast-feeding. If the infant exhibits poor growth, alternate breast and bottle feeds with MCT formula feeds, to provide approximately half the infant's requirements from MCT formula, i.e. 75–90 mL/kg/day.

Using a modular feed

Infants with decompensated liver disease may require modular feeding in which fluid, sodium or protein is separately prescribed. Used when a calorie dense (up to 2 kcal/mL)/low volume feed is required.

Weaning diet

Weaning as normal at 6 months except for the use of MCT formula mixed in with dried baby foods and cereals.

Further reading

Hartley J, Davenport M, Kelly D. Biliary atresia. *Lancet* 2009;374:1704–1713

Key web links

BSPGHAN guidelines for investigation of conjugated jaundice:
http://www.bspghan.org.uk/document/liver/Investigationof
NeonatalConjugatedhyperbilirubinaemia.pdf
Information for families on all causes of cholestasis:
http://www.childliverdisease.org/content/414/Liver-Diseases
-Jaundice-in-Babies
NICE guidelines for neonatal cholestasis: http://guidance.nice.org.uk/
CG98/Guidance/pdf/English; pages 14–29 provide phototherapy
charts

The acutely unwell infant

Acute liver dysfunction or liver failure in a baby should be investigated and treated at a specialist paediatric liver unit. Acute liver dysfunction may present in the newborn period secondary to a metabolic disease or an intrauterine infection, or may develop at weaning.

Important features from history

- Consanguinity
- Affected siblings
- Miscarriages
- Pregnancy and birth history
- Dietary and fasting history
- Difficulty in feeding or vomiting: may indicate encephalopathy in neonates

Clinical assessment and investigations

- Liver and spleen size
- Tachypnoea
- Abnormal neurology
- Intercurrent infection
- Urine in some urea cycle disorders has an unusual odour

Algorithm 18.1 and Table 18.1, Table 18.2 and Table 18.3 summarise the differential diagnosis, investigations, treatment and outcome. See Chapter 30 for management of liver failure.

Practical Approach to Paediatric Gastroenterology, Hepatology and Nutrition, First Edition.
Deirdre Kelly, Ronald Bremner, Jane Hartley, and Diana Flynn.
© 2014 John Wiley & Sons, Ltd. Published 2014 by John Wiley & Sons, Ltd.

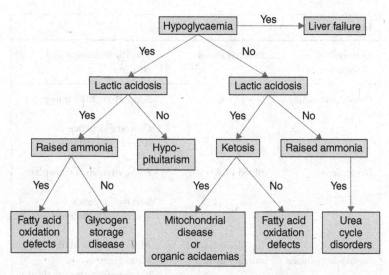

Algorithm 18.1 Investigations for suspected metabolic disease

Table 18.1 Differential diagnosis, investigations, treatment and outcome of acute liver disease presenting in neonates

Differential diagnosis	Investigations	Specific treatment and outcome
Herpes simplex	Blood and urine PCR Immunofluorescence of vesicle swabs	Aciclovir (20 mg/kg 8 hourly for 14 days) Multisystem disease with high mortality
Adenovirus	Blood PCR	Cidofovir (5 mg/kg weekly, requires pre-treatment with probenicid and hyperhydration) Outcome depends on severity of viral infection
ECHO virus	Stool PCR	Supportive, liver transplant Survival depends on severity of viral infection
		(Continued)

Table 18.1 (*Continued*)

Differential diagnosis	Investigations	Specific treatment and outcome
Coxsacchie virus	Stool PCR	Supportive, liver transplant Outcome depends on severity of viral infection
Parvovirus	Blood PCR	Supportive, liver transplant Survival depends on severity of viral infection
Neonatal haemochromatosis	Lip biopsy: iron in salivary glands MRI T2 images: high iron content of pancreas and liver as compared to spleen	Antioxidant cocktail, plamapheresis and immunoglobulins (medical management only effective in mild cases), liver transplantation
Mitochondrial disease	High blood and cerebrospinal fluid (CSF) lactate Muscle biopsy (fat droplets and ragged red fibres) Mitochondrial DNA from blood, liver or muscle EEG	Multisystem progressive life-limiting disease Liver transplant is contraindicated Palliative care
Galactosaemia	Reducing substances in urine, galactose-1-phosphate uridyl transferase	Lactose free diet Long-term stabilisation on diet, but learning difficulties and infertility are common

Table 18.1 (*Continued*)

Differential diagnosis	Investigations	Specific treatment and outcome
Urea cycle disorders	Raised ammonia Plasma amino acids	Emergency management of hyperammonaemia: see Red flags Hepatocyte transplant as a rescue therapy Maintenance treatment: protein restricted diet Liver transplant for complications Most neonates die at first presentation or have neurological abnormalities Lifelong risk of hyperammonaemia coma
Fatty acid oxidation defects	Acyl carnitines, low carnitine, lactic acidosis, raised ammonia, raised creatinine kinase	Avoid fasting using nasogastric feeding and cornstarch 60% mortality at presentation In those who survive, long-term outcome is good
Organic acidaemias	Acidosis, hyperammonaemia, urine organic acids	Emergency treatment of hyperammonaemia (see Red flags) Correct hypoglycaemia and acidosis, carnitine (200 mg/kg/day) and metronidazole (20 mg/kg/day) in the acute illness Maintenance with low protein, high calorie diet

(*Continued*)

Table 18.1 (*Continued*)

Differential diagnosis	Investigations	Specific treatment and outcome
		Vulnerable to the development of neurological disease, stroke, basal ganglia changes and developmental delay in childhood. Liver transplant in early childhood may prevent neurological deterioration.
Carbohydrate deficient glycoprotein (CDG) defect	Transferrin electrophoresis DNA	Supportive therapy Mannose in CDG Ib Survival beyond 2 years is rare In those with CDG Ib, there is progressive liver disease
Familial haemophagocytic lymphohistiocytosis	Raised triglycerides, low fibrinogen and coagulopathy, low albumin and sodium DNA (five different genes)	Chemotherapy (steroids and etoposide) but relapse is common Stem cell transplant may be curative Liver transplant is contraindicated
Glycogen storage disease	Low blood glucose, acidosis, raised triglycerides, raised uric acid DNA	Prevent hypoglycaemia with frequent feeding, overnight nasogastric feeding or cornstarch Liver transplant for development of liver adenomas or poor metabolic control

EEG, electroencephalogram; PCR, polymerase chain reaction.

Table 18.2 Differential diagnosis investigations, treatment and outcome of acute liver disease presenting later in infancy

Differential diagnosis	Investigations	Specific treatment and outcome
Tyrosinaemia type 1	Urinary succinyl acetone elevated, raised alpha-fetoprotein (40 000–70 000 kU/L), increased plasma tyrosine, phenylalanine, methionine, proximal renal tubular dysfunction, cardiomyopathy, rickets	NTBC (nitisinone) (1 mg/kg/day) with dietary restriction of phenylalanine and tyrosine Without treatment there is an 80% mortality rate and high risk of hepatocellular carcinoma NTBC stabilises the clinical features within a few days and liver transplant is rarely indicated
Glycogen storage disease	See Table 18.1	
Hereditary fructose intolerance (presents at weaning with introduction of fructose-containing foods)	Enzyme deficiency in liver or intestinal mucosa, DNA, hypoglycaemia, lactic acidosis, amino acid uria, anaemia, thrombocytopenia	Exclude fructose, sucrose and sorbitol from the diet for life

Table 18.3 Differential diagnosis, investigations, treatment and outcome of acute liver disease presenting with neonatal ascites or hydrops

Differential diagnosis	Investigations	Specific treatment and outcome
Lysosomal storage disease (Niemann Pick C, Gaucher's and Wolman's disease)	Glucocerebrosidase (from leucocytes or fibroblasts), storage cells in bone marrow or liver biopsy, DNA, adrenal calcification in Wolman's disease	Gaucher's: recombinant enzyme therapy with good long-term survival in type 1 (most common) Niemann Pick C: enzyme replacement, palliation due to progressive neurological deterioration within the first 3 decades (see Information: Neimann Pick C type 1) Wolman's: supportive therapy, liver transplant for liver failure, enzyme replacement therapy Death in infancy is common
Cytomegalovirus (CMV)	Urine and blood PCR	Usually self-limiting but ganciclovir (5 mg/kg 12 hourly) may be useful in liver failure, for retinitis and to prevent hearing loss
Toxoplasma	Serology	Spiramycin (50 mg/kg 12 hourly) may prevent progression

Table 18.3 (*Continued*)

Differential diagnosis	Investigations	Specific treatment and outcome
Syphilis	Venereal disease research laboratory (VDRL) test and antitreponemal antibodies	Benzylpenicillin (25 mg/kg 12 hourly)
Tyrosinaemia	See Table 18.2	
Mitochondrial disease	See Table 18.1	
Carbohydrate deficient glycoprotein syndrome	See Table 18.1	
Heart failure	Echocardiography	Diuretics, corrective cardiac treatment
Haemangioendothelioma	Ultrasound scan, echocardiography	Diuretics, steroids, embolisation of feeding vessel, liver transplant
	Haemolysis, MR angiography	

PCR, polymerase chain reaction.

Initial investigations to establish if there is liver failure
- Prothrombin time
- Blood glucose
- Split bilirubin
- Transaminases
- Albumin (ALB)

Management
- Stop feeds
- Give IV fluids until galactosaemia, tyrosinaemia and urea cycle disorders are excluded
- Manage acute liver failure if coagulation abnormal (PT raised) (see Chapter 30)
- Maintain blood sugars in the normal range with intravenous glucose

Specific management

Neonatal haemochromatosis

This is a liver alloimmune disease resulting in iron overload that spares the reticuloendothelial system. The diagnosis is based on iron deposition in liver and extrahepatic organs, such as the pancreas and brain.

Red flags: Pitfalls in interpreting ferritin levels

A raised ferritin (>1000 µg/L; normal range 32–233 µg/L) is indicative of neonatal haemochromatosis but may be raised in liver necrosis, such as herpes simplex, and is not diagnostic.

An antioxidant cocktail may stabilise the disease if mild or enable survival to liver transplant:
- N-acetylcysteine: oral 140 mg/kg/day on day 1 followed by 70 mg/kg/day for up to 3 weeks. Give in three divided doses
- Selenium: IV 3 µg/kg/day over 24 hours (unless on parenteral nutrition)
- Alpha-tocopheryl acetate: orally 25 mg/kg/day for 6 weeks
- Prostaglandin E1 (Alprotadil): IV 0.4 µg/kg/hour, which can be increased to 0.6 µg/kg/hour if tolerated
- Desferrioxamine: IV 30 mg/kg/day over 8 hours until serum ferritin is <500 µg/L

Plasmapharesis to reduce the level of circulating antibody followed by immunoglobulin infusions may also be beneficial.

Liver transplantation is usually required.

In subsequent pregnancies women should be advised to have immunoglobulin

infusions from 18 weeks' gestation to prevent recurrence.

Mitochondrial disease

This multisystem, life-limiting disease presents with acute liver failure. It should be suspected in any infant with high lactate after resuscitation.

It may present in later childhood with developmental delay and epilepsy. There are numerous mitochondrial defects. Mitochondrial DNA from blood and muscle may identify the metabolic defect and enable counselling and prenatal testing.

Neonatal herpes simplex

Herpes simplex is a multisystem disease that may be fatal. All neonates with liver failure should receive aciclovir until the results of investigations are known.

Red flags: Management of hyperammonaemia

- Stop protein
- If ammonia >200 μmol/L:
  - IV 10% dextrose
  - Sodium benzoate:
    - Loading dose 250 mg/kg
    - Continuous infusion 250 mg/kg/day
  - Arginine in 10% dextrose:
    - Loading dose 350 mg/kg over 2 hours
    - Continuous infusion 350 mg/kg/day
- If ammonia >400 μmol/L or rising:
  - Dialysis
  - Continuous infusion of sodium phenylbutyrate 250 mg/kg/day
  - Repeated loading dose of arginine and sodium benzoate

The infant with splenomegaly

The spleen should not be palpable so splenomegaly requires further investigation.

History

- Family history, consanguinity, neonatal deaths or miscarriages
- Failure to thrive or weight loss
- Previous illnesses or hypoglycaemia
- Jaundice
- Easy bruising/epistaxis

Differential diagnosis

- Infection:
  - Congenital infection [rubella, cytomegalovirus (CMV), toxoplasmosis]
  - Epstein–Barr virus (EBV)
  - CMV (acquired)
- Haematological:
  - Sickle cell disease
  - Thalassaemia
  - Autoimmune thrombocytopenia or haemolytic anaemia
- Portal hypertension: any cause of chronic liver disease or extrahepatic portal venous obstruction
- Malignancy:
  - Leukaemia
  - Lymphoma

Practical Approach to Paediatric Gastroenterology, Hepatology and Nutrition, First Edition.
Deirdre Kelly, Ronald Bremner, Jane Hartley, and Diana Flynn.

- Storage disorder: Niemann Pick C, Wolman's disease
- Peroxisomal biogenesis disorders: Zellweger's syndrome

Investigations

- Blood:
  - FBC, blood film, reticulocyte count: haematological or hypersplenism
  - LFTs, prothrombin: acute or chronic liver disease
  - Glucose, lactate, urate, free fatty acids, 3-hydroxybutyrate, cholesterol and triglycerides, creatine kinase: glycogen storage disease
  - Sphingomyelinase: Nieman Pick type A
  - Very long chain fatty acids (VLCFA): Zellweger's
  - Hepatitis A serology, CMV and EBV PCR
  - Lysosomal acid lipase for Wolman's disease
- Urine: vanillymandelic acid in neuroblastoma
- Liver biopsy: histology – storage cells, although in neonates they are not often seen, or glycogen
- Ultrasound:
  - Portal hypertension: varices, small portal vein, high hepatic resistive index
  - Enlarged lymph nodes in lymphoma or masses along the sympathetic chain in neuroblastoma
  - Cystic malformation of the kidneys and brain in Zellweger's syndrome
- X-ray:
  - Adrenal calcification in Wolman's disease
  - Epiphyseal calcification in Zellweger's syndrome
- Bone marrow aspirate: storage cells of Neiman Pick C
- Genetic investigation: Niemann Pick C, Wolman's disease, Zellweger's syndrome
- Fibroblast studies: Niemann Pick C (Filipin test), Wolman's disease

---

Information: Neimann Pick C type 1

This is an abnormality of cholesterol esterification caused by mutations in NPC1 or NPC2.

Presentation is with prolonged jaundice, hepatomegaly and marked splenomegaly and foetal ascites. The liver disease resolves but splenomegaly increases.

Developmental delay, ataxia, convulsions and vertical supranuclear ophthalmoplegia develop within one to three decades. Most die in childhood or early adolescence from pneumonia.

Neonatal liver disease may be fatal, but cholestasis may improve. Enzyme replacement therapy is now available for those who develop early signs of neurological progression (Miglustat). Liver or bone marrow transplant is not curative.

Further reading

Shanmugam NP, Bansal S, Greenough A, Verma A, Dhawan A. Neonatal liver failure: aetiologies and management–state of the art. *Eur J Pediatr* 2011;170: 573–581

Key web links

http://www.climb.org.uk/
www.neonatalhemochromatosis.org

The infant with a hepatic cause for abdominal distension

CHAPTER 20

Causes

Possible hepatic causes of abdominal distension are:
- Fluid: ascites
- Tumour: abdominal distension may be the presenting feature (Figure 20.1)
- Organomegaly due to liver disease, storage disorders or splenomegaly

History

- Liver disease
- Developmental delay
- Dysmorphism
- Abdominal pain
- Easy bruising
- Weight loss

Hepatoblastoma is associated with hemihypertrophy, a family history of familial adenomatous polyposis (FAP) due to mutations in the *APC* gene and precocious puberty

Examination

- Ascites will be identified by shifting dullness and a fluid thrill
- Organomegaly, dysmorphism, hemihypertrophy, ear folds in Beckwith–Weidermann syndrome
- There may be peripheral stigmata of chronic liver disease as the underlying pathology of portal hypertension with splenomegaly

---

Practical Approach to Paediatric Gastroenterology, Hepatology and Nutrition, First Edition.
Deirdre Kelly, Ronald Bremner, Jane Hartley, and Diana Flynn.
© 2014 John Wiley & Sons, Ltd. Published 2014 by John Wiley & Sons, Ltd.

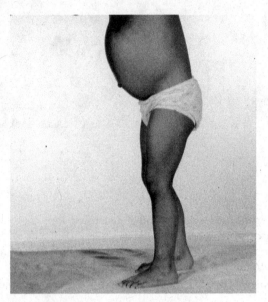

Figure 20.1 Liver enlargement due to a hepatic tumour.

Differential diagnosis

- Ascites: chronic liver disease of any cause (may be sudden-onset ascites following a variceal bleed or sepsis):
  - Heart failure
  - Budd–Chiari syndrome
- Neonatal ascites: see Table 18.3
- Malignancy: hepatoblastoma, neuroblastoma, haemangioendothelioma (see Chapter 23), mesenchymal hamartoma
- Storage disease:
  - Neimann Pick A, B or C
  - Glycogen storage disease

Investigations

- Liver biochemistry: aspartate transaminase (AST), alanine transaminase (ALT) and bilirubin are elevated in chronic liver disease and storage disorders. They are normal in hepatoblastoma
- Liver synthetic markers: albumin and clotting may be abnormal in chronic liver disease. May be normal in late presentation of Niemann Pick C
- FBC: platelets may be reduced in hypersplenism; abnormal morphology of lymphocytes in Wolman's disease; thrombocytosis with hepatoblastomas

Specific blood investigations

- High lactate and lipids for glycogen storage disease
- Tumour markers: alpha-fetoprotein (AFP) is elevated in hepatoblastoma (NB: AFP is high in neonates and falls with age)
- Ascitic tap: essential to diagnose bacterial peritonitis in a child with ascites and fever (see Chapter 25)
- Urine: catecholamines (VMAs) raised in neuroblastoma, oligosaccharides raised in mucolipidoses and mucopolysaccharides raised in mucopolysaccharidosis
- Abdominal X-ray: adrenal calcification of Wolman's disease
- Ultrasound: to identify mass lesion within the liver, confirm organomegaly and mark a suitable spot for an ascitic tap
- CT or MRI scan: tumour morphology and stage, and identify extrahepatic metastases
- Histology: to confirm grade and diagnosis of tumour; identify storage cells
- Bone marrow: to identify lysosomal storage cells
- Fibroblast culture: to identify enzyme deficiency in lysosomal storage diseases
- DNA: *NPC1* and 2 gene mutations for Neimann Pick C, gene transcription abnormality in Beckwith–Weidermann syndrome

Management

Ascites

- Diuretics: spironolactone (3 mg/kg) takes 2–3 days before effect and if resistant, furosemide (1–2 mg/kg)
- Albumin replacement: 5 ml/kg 20% human albumin solution (HAS) given over 4 hours with furosemide (1 mg/kg)
- Paracentesis: tense ascites with dyspnoea or pain, percutaneous removal replacing half volume with 4.5% HAS

Information: Hepatic malignancy

Hepatoblastoma is the most common hepatic tumour in those under 5 years of age.

It is associated with:
- Beckwith–Weidermann syndrome
- Wilms' tumours
- Familial adenomatous polyposis (*FAP* gene)
- Hemihypertrophy

(Continued)

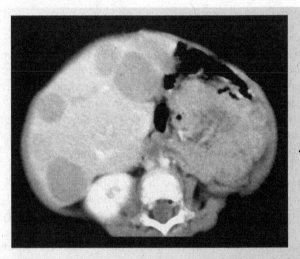

Figure 20.2 CT scan showing tumour in both lobes of the liver and which is therefore unresectable. (Source: Diseases of the Liver and Biliary System in Children, Third Edition. Edited by Deirdre Kelly. Reproduced with permission of John Wiley & Sons Ltd.)

- Gardner's syndrome
- Trisomies
- Fetal alcohol syndrome

Hepatoblastoma is graded according to the extent of liver involvement (Figure 20.2) and grade determines the chemotherapy regimen (SIOPEL-3), the potential for resection or the need for liver transplantation. Treatment response is monitored using AFP.

Hepatocellular carcinoma (HCC)

Rare in childhood but may develop with cirrhosis, untreated tyrosinaemia, hepatitis B and C and progressive familial intrahepatic cholestasis (PFIC) type 2. It presents with abdominal pain and/or mass, or an increase in AFP. It is poorly responsive to chemotherapy, but liver transplantation may be an option if there is no extrahepatic disease. HCC screening using AFP and MRI scan is required in those with a high risk.

Lysosomal storage disorders

Present with hepatomegaly and splenomegaly with or without neurological involvement at the time of presentation (Table 20.1). Of the lysosomal storage diseases, the hepatic manifestations are more common in Gaucher's, Neimann Pick C, cholesterol ester storage disease and Wolman's disease.

Table 20.1 Clinical features, investigations, management and outcome of lysosomal storage disorders

Disease group	Specific disease	Diagnosis	Management	Outcome
Sphingolipid	Niemann Pick (NP) A, B, C	Hepatosplenomegaly	Type A: palliation	Type A: fatal in infancy
		Identify storage cells from liver, bone marrow or duodenum	Type B: management of respiratory symptoms	Type B: long-term survival with huge hepatosplenomegaly
		Mutation studies:		Lung involvement may be severe
		NPA&B: *SMPD1*	Type C: see Information: Neimann Pick C type 1	
		NPC: *NPC1* and 2		Type C: see Information: Neimann Pick C type 1
		Fibroblast: Filipin staining		
	Gaucher's disease types 1, 2 and 3	Hepatosplenomegaly, hypersplenism, glucocerebrosidase level in leucocytes, Gaucher cells in bone marrow, increased ACE	Type 1 and 3 recombinant enzyme therapy. Type 2 is supportive only	Type 1 and 3 can live normal lives with treatment. Type 2 is fatal in infancy with progressive neurological involvement.
		Mutation analysis		

(Continued)

Table 20.1 (*Continued*)

Disease group	Specific disease	Diagnosis	Management	Outcome
	Wolman's disease	Hepatosplenomegaly, diarrhoea, adrenal calcification, vacuolated lymphocytes, storage cells in bone marrow, liver or duodenum, hypertriglyceridaemia, hypercholesterolaemia	Reduce lipid with low fat diet and cholestyramine	See Table 18.3
			Supportive	Death in childhood
Mucolipidosis	Mucolipidosis type 1	Hepatosplenomegaly, cherry red spot, psychomotor retardation, seizures	Palliative	Death in infancy although mild cases can survive into adulthood
Mucopolysaccharidosis	Hurler's (MPS1)	Hepatosplenomegaly, coarse facial features, psychomotor retardation, mucopolysaccharide in urine	Palliative	Death by 8–10 years
	Sialic acid	Hepatosplenomegaly, coarse facial features, psychomotor retardation, cardiomyopathy mucopolysaccharide in urine	Palliative	Death by 1–5 years

Key web links

http://emedicine.medscape.com/article/986802-treatment#a1127
http://www.cancer.gov/cancertopics/pdq/treatment/childliver/
  HealthProfessional/page1

The older child with jaundice

CHAPTER 21

Important features from history

- Contact with infection
- Tiredness, anorexia and vague abdominal pain
- Autoimmune conditions/autoimmune disease in the family (coeliac disease, diabetes, hypothyroidism)
- Ulcerative colitis: associated with the development of sclerosing cholangitis
- Deterioration in school work and slurring of words: indicative of Wilson's disease
- Recent introduction of new medication including antibiotics
- Weight loss, pallor, bruising may be indicative of malignancy

Differential diagnosis

Jaundice in an older child may be the first sign of chronic liver disease (Table 21.1). It is important to exclude Gilbert's syndrome which presents in teenagers with unconjugated jaundice (see Algorithm 17.1). Cases should be discussed with a liver paediatric liver centre.

Management

- Supportive management for all conditions with fat-soluble vitamins,
- Nutritional support and antipruritics
- Autoimmune hepatitis: see Information: Autoimmune hepatitis I and II
- Sclerosing cholangitis: high dose ursodeoxycholic acid 30 mg/kg/day (± steroids or therapy for inflammatory bowel disease as required)
- Wilson's disease: see Information: Wilson's disease

Practical Approach to Paediatric Gastroenterology, Hepatology and Nutrition, First Edition. Deirdre Kelly, Ronald Bremner, Jane Hartley, and Diana Flynn.
© 2014 John Wiley & Sons, Ltd. Published 2014 by John Wiley & Sons, Ltd.

Table 21.1 Differential diagnosis and investigations of older children with jaundice

Differential diagnosis	Investigation
Acute viral infection A, B, E, Epstein–Barr virus (EBV)	Serology, RNA or DNA
Seronegative hepatitis	By exclusion
Autoimmune hepatitis (AIH) See Information: Autoimmune hepatitis I and II	Type 1 AIH: antinuclear antibody (ANA) and smooth muscle antibody (SMA) positive
	Type 2 AIH: Liver–kidney–microsomal (LKM) positive
	IgG significantly raised
	Complement C3 and C4 low
	Histology: plasma cell infiltrate of the portal tract which spills into the surrounding parenchyma (interface hepatitis), varying degrees of parenchymal collapse and fibrosis
Sclerosing cholangitis	pANCA positive
	Ultrasound: gallbladder enlarged and the bile ducts may be dilated and irregular
	Magnetic resonance cholangiopancreatogram (MRCP): beading of bile ducts
	Histology: onion skin fibrosis around the bile duct
Wilson's disease See Information: Wilson's disease	Raised serum copper
	Low caeruloplasmin
	ANA and SMA occasionally positive
	Mildly raised IgG
	Haemolytic anaemia
	Low alkaline phosphatase
	DNA: *ATP7B* mutations

(*Continued*)

Table 21.1 (*Continued*)

Differential diagnosis	Investigation
	Urine: 24-hour urine copper followed by a 24-hour urine collection after penicillamine at 0 and 12 hours if raised is very indicative of Wilson's disease
	MRI changes in basal ganglia
	Ophthalmology: Kaiser–Fleisher rings Figure 21.1 Histology: micro and macro vesicular steatosis with varying degrees of portal inflammation and fibrosis; Mallory bodies, lipofuscin and copper will also be seen; liver for copper >250 μg/g dry weight (normal <55) is indicative
Alpha-1-antitrypsin deficiency	Alpha-1-antitrypsin level and phenotype
Benign recurrent intrahepatic cholestasis (BRIC)	*ATP8B1*, *ABCB11*, *ABCB4* mutations
Drug-induced liver disease (DILD)	See Information: Drug-induced liver disease
Leukaemia, lymphoma	Effects on bone marrow
	Histology: leukaemic infiltrate

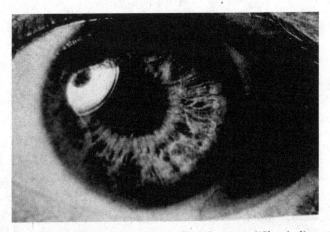

Figure 21.1 Kaiser–Fleischer rings are usually only seen in Wilson's disease after the age of 7 years.

Information: Autoimmune hepatitis I and II

Clinical features

Variable presentation, occurs at any age:
- Malaise
- Intermittent jaundice with abdominal pain and anorexia
- Splenomegaly
- Acute liver failure
  Associated with other autoimmune disorders.

Management
- Prednisolone 2mg/kg (max 40mg) daily (with omeprazole 10–20mg daily)
- Wean with weekly reductions as biochemistry improves
- Add azathioprine 1mg/kg when LFTs are normal
- Check response and bone marrow suppression with weekly blood tests for a month and then 3 monthly

Indications for transplant
- Fulminant hepatic failure
- Complications of cirrhosis
- Failure of medical therapy/intolerable side-effects
  25% recurrence of AIH following transplant.

Information: Drug-induced liver disease

Clinical features
- May develop any time after therapy
- Presents with non-specific symptoms: fever, rash and eosinophilia
- Liver involvement ranges from abnormal transaminases to liver failure.

Diagnosis
- Temporal related to ingestion of drug
- Exclude other causes of liver disease
- Histology: necrosis with inflammatory cell infiltrate in acute drug-induced liver disease, cholestasis and bile duct injury; granulomatous changes with carbamazepine; features similar to autoimmune hepatitis, fatty change, fibrosis or sinusoidal dilatation in chronic disease

Management
- Withdrawal of the drug
- N-acetylcystine in paracetamol toxicity
- Transplant for acute liver failure

Information: Wilson's disease

Wilson's disease is an autosomal recessive disorder (*ATPB7*) of copper handling in the liver resulting in accumulation of toxic copper within the liver and the brain.

Clinical features
- Younger children present with liver disease, such as hepatomegaly, jaundice, acute or chronic hepatitis, liver failure, portal hypertension and decompensated cirrhosis
- Teenagers and adults present with neurological problems, such as abnormal speech, incoordination, deterioration in school work, intention tremor

Management
- Chelation therapy with zinc acetate (fewer side-effects) (dose 1–6 years 25 mg twice daily; >6 years, if <57 kg 25 mg three times daily; >57 kg 50 mg three times daily) or penicillamine, but this may cause many side-effects including deterioration in neurological function
- Liver transplant for acute liver failure, or non-response to therapy. Using the Wilson's disease score may help determine need for transplantation in acute liver failure (further reading)

Red flags: Common drugs causing liver disease

- Cholestasis:
  - Co-amoxiclav
  - Erythromycin
  - Sulphonamides
  - Ketoconazole
  - Carbamazepine
- Hepatocellular inflammation:
  - Paracetamol
  - Non-steroidal anti-inflammatories
  - Cephalosporin
  - Tetracyclines cause fatty infiltration
  - Erythromycin
  - Ketoconazole
  - Carbamazepine
  - Phenytoin
  - Isoniazid

- Damage to bile ducts:
  - Flucloxacillin
  - Tetracycline
  - Ampicillin/amoxicillin
  - Co-amixoclav

Further reading

European Association for Study of Liver. EASL Clinical Practice Guidelines: Wilson's disease. *J Hepatol* 2012;56:671–685

Hennes EM, Zeniya M, Czaja AJ, *et al*. Simplified criteria for the diagnosis of autoimmune hepatitis. *Hepatology* 2008;48:169–176

Murray KF, Hadzic N, Wirth S, Bassett M, Kelly D. Drug-related hepatotoxicity and acute liver failure. *J Pediatr Gastroenterol Nutr* 2008;47:395–405

Key web link

www.aasld.org/practiceguidelines/Documents/AIH2010.PDF

The older child who is acutely unwell

CHAPTER 22

Important features from history

- Any previous medical history and medications
- Deterioration in school performance or changes in speech
- Developmental delay or neurological deterioration
- Known prothrombotic disorder
- Previous episodes of jaundice
- Recent sodium valproate

Differential diagnosis

The medical history is helpful in directing investigation and differential diagnosis (Table 22.1). In children with seronegative hepatitis with no significant past medical history there is a poor chance of recovery without liver transplant.

Practical Approach to Paediatric Gastroenterology, Hepatology and Nutrition, First Edition.
Deirdre Kelly, Ronald Bremner, Jane Hartley, and Diana Flynn.
© 2014 John Wiley & Sons, Ltd. Published 2014 by John Wiley & Sons, Ltd.

Table 22.1 Differential diagnosis, specific investigations and management of a child with acute liver dysfunction

Differential diagnosis	Investigations	Management
Hepatitis viruses A,B,E, EBV, CMV, parvovirus	Viral serology HAV RNA, HBV DNA, HEV RNA	Resolve with conservative management
Seronegative hepatitis	Aplastic anaemia may occur with seronegative hepatitis pre or post transplant. There is a high mortality rate	Supportive therapy. 70% require liver transplant
Autoimmune hepatitis type I or II	see Table 21.1	See Chapter 21, Information: Autoimmune hepatitis I and II
Wilson's disease	Low alkaline phosphatase	Zinc acetate as a chelation agent
	Haemolysis	Acute presentation may require super urgent transplant
	Mildly raised immunoglobulins	
	ANA may be raised	See Chapter 21, Information: Wilson's disease
	Urine copper estimation	
Metabolic conditions, e.g. glycogen storage disease (GSD)	Hypoglycaemia, increased urate and lactate	Management of hypoglycaemia with corn starch
	Ultrasound: hyperechoic due to fat accumulation	In GSD type 1 neutropenia may require granulocyte colony-stimulating factor
Mitochondrial disease, e.g. *POLG* mutations	Raised lactate	No proven therapy

(Continued)

Table 22.1 (*Continued*)

Differential diagnosis	Investigations	Management
Paracetamol overdose	Raised paracetamol levels	See Information: Paracetamol overdose
Drug-induced liver disease	History of drug ingestion	Exclusion of causative agent
	Liver biopsy may be diagnostic	
	See Chapter 21, Information: Drug-induced liver disease	
Vascular anomalies such as Budd–Chiari syndrome	Protein C and S, factor V Leiden, antithrombin III deficiency, factor II prothrombin gene mutation, antiphospholipid antibodies	Refer to specialised centre for stenting of the hepatic veins using a transjugular intrahepatic portosystemic shunt (TiPPS) (artificial hepatic shunt inserted percutaneously via neck veins) and formal anticoagulation
	Ultrasound: to identify venous outflow obstruction	

Information: Paracetamol overdose

- Determine from the history:
  - Time of overdose and whether it was staggered
  - Any other drugs or alcohol taken
  - Significant past medical history
- At 4 hours following the overdose take blood for:
  - Paracetamol level
  - LFT
  - Clotting
  - U&E
  - Venous gas
  - Blood sugar

- If a significant overdose, delayed presentation or staggered overdose, commence treatment before taking the paracetamol levels

Treatment
- N-acetylcysteine is a very potent antidote [for dose see http://www2 .pharmweb.net/pwmirror/pwy/paracetamol/chart.html
  Ranitidine: intravenous 3mg/kg three times daily
- Vitamin K: 10mg
Clotting should be monitored 12 hourly or until the trend is stable or improving.
  Criteria for referral to a paediatric liver transplant centre include:
- INR >2.5
- Acidosis
- Renal dysfunction
- Encephalopathy
- Hypoglycaemia
  Stop N-acetylcysteine when the PT is <18 (INR<1.5).

Information: Seronegative hepatitis

- Most common cause of acute liver worldwide
- Diagnosis made by exclusion
- 70% mortality rate without transplantation
- Aplastic anaemia may develop pre or post transplant

Management

See Chapter 30.

Further reading

Ferner RE, Dear JW, Bateman DN. Management of paracetamol poisoning. *BMJ* 2011;342:1– 9

Sundaram SS, Alonso EM, Narkewicz MR, Zhang S, Squires RH; Pediatric Acute Liver Failure Study Group. Characterization and outcomes of young infants with acute liver failure. *J Pediatr* 2011;159:813–818.e1

Key web links

http://gut.bmj.com/content/45/suppl_6/VI1.full
http://www.ninds.nih.gov/disorders/alpersdisease/alpersdisease .htm

The older child with hepatic causes of abdominal distension

Abdominal distension may be progression of a known disease, e.g. fibrocystic disease, or the initial presentation, e.g. hepatocellular carcinoma (HCC).

Important features from history

- Family history of blood clots
- Recent commencement of oral contraceptive pill
- Poor weight gain or weight loss in tumours
- Diabetes
- Renal dysfunction or failure in fibrocystic disease

Differential diagnosis

- Fibrocystic disease
- Budd–Chiari syndrome Menon KV, 2004
- Hepatocellular carcinoma (HCC)
- Uncontrolled diabetes

Presenting features

Abdominal distension may be due to:
- Fluid: ascites extensive in Budd–Chiari
- Organs: enlarged liver, spleen and kidney in fibrocystic disease
- Hepatomegaly (and/or splenomegaly): Budd–Chiari, uncontrolled diabetes (secondary to glycogen and fat) or cystic fibrosis liver disease (CFLD)
- Tumour: liver tumours

Practical Approach to Paediatric Gastroenterology, Hepatology and Nutrition, First Edition.
Deirdre Kelly, Ronald Bremner, Jane Hartley, and Diana Flynn.

Investigations

- Biochemistry: Raised transaminases in Budd–Chiari (>1000 IU/L in acute disease)
- Cholangitis in fibrocystic disease, HCC and uncontrolled diabetes
- Renal function: renal failure in fibrocystic disease with renal involvement
- Tumour markers: alpha-fetoprotein (AFP) is raised in 50% of HCC
- Haematology:
  - Polycythaemia in HCC
  - Thrombocythemia in hypersplenism in fibrocystic disease, cirrhosis or CFLD
  - Clotting: elevated PT in Budd–Chiari syndrome. There may be an underlying malignancy or prothrombotic condition in Budd–Chiari syndrome. Protein C, protein S, lupus anticoagulant, prothrombin III, factor V Leiden should be measured. There may be hepatic decompensation in fibrocystic disease complicated by cholangitis or in CFLD
- Bone marrow: to identify malignancy (leukaemia or myeloproliferative disease) which may be the underlying cause of Budd–Chiari
- Ultrasound:
  - Tumour mass within the liver; poor flow seen in the hepatic veins and hypertrophy of caudate lobe in Budd–Chiari
  - Liver will be hyperreflective due to fatty infiltration in diabetes
  - Irregular shape with portal hypertension in fibrocystic disease
- CT scan:
  - Staging of tumour and extrahepatic disease
  - CT angiography for flow in the hepatic veins in Budd–Chiari
- Magnetic resonance cholangiopancreatogram (MRCP): to identify biliary involvement in fibrocystic disease
- Liver biopsy under CT or ultrasound guidance: essential for tumour histology

Management

Budd-Chiari

- Medical treatment of ascites
- Anticoagulation with heparin/warfarin (investigations for procoagulant conditions should be sent prior to commencing heparin and warfarin)
- Stenting of hepatic veins by interventional radiology
- Liver transplant may be required if there is hepatic failure or shunting is unsuccessful, but there is a risk of recurrence following transplant if there is a procoagulant tendency

Fibrocystic disease

- Liver function is usually normal, but therapy is required for portal hypertension and recurrent cholangitis
- Liver and kidney transplantation if significant renal failure

Diabetes

- Tighter control of diabetes

Hepatocellular carcinoma

- 50% of cases will respond to chemotherapy but the overall 5-year survival is 28%
- Response is monitored by CT scan and AFP levels
- Liver transplant may be indicated in small tumours following chemotherapy

---

Information: Fibrocystic disease

- Ductal plate malformations are due to an abnormality of primary cilia (ciliopathies). Renal disease may be the presenting feature causing morbidity Gunay-Aygun M, 2009
- Liver complications are hepatomegaly, cholangitis and portal hypertension
- Renal transplant is often needed prior to the development of significant liver complications but a combined transplant has the best long-term outcome

---

Further reading

Gunay-Aygun M. Liver and kidney disease in ciliopathies. *Am J Med Genet C Semin Med Genet* 2009;151C:296–306

Menon KV, Shah V, Kamath PS. The Budd–Chiari syndrome. *N Engl J Med* 2004;350:578–585

Chronic liver disease: itching

Itching or pruritis is a common symptom in chronic biliary diseases. The exact mechanism is unknown but it may be due to build-up of toxins not excreted due to cholestasis. It is distressing, prevents sleep and is detrimental to development. Children are usually, but not always jaundiced. Examination reveals excoriation marks with dry skin. It is difficult to treat effectively but may improve with time in young children.

In younger children it is most commonly seen in cholestatic conditions:
- Biliary atresia (see Chapter 17, Information: Biliary atresia)
- Progressive familial intrahepatic cholestasis (see Chapter 17, Information: Low GGT cholestasis)
- Alagille syndrome (see Chapter 17, Information: Alagille syndrome)

In older children it is seen in:
- Infectious hepatitis
- Obstructive jaundice, e.g. gallstones
- Benign recurrent intrahepatic cholestasis (BRIC)
- Sclerosing cholangitis: this is a disease of the intra- and extra-hepatic bile ducts, which is associated with ulcerative colitis and autoimmune liver disease. Ursodeoxycholic acid is the only effective treatment. Long-term follow-up to identify progression of liver disease and determine the timing for transplantation if necessary
- Chronic rejection post transplant

Important features from history

- Previous chronic liver disease or transplant
- Inflammatory bowel disease or bowel symptoms
- Recent ingestion of oral contraception containing oestrogen
- Family history of jaundice in pregnancy or on oral contraceptive pill

Practical Approach to Paediatric Gastroenterology, Hepatology and Nutrition, First Edition.
Deirdre Kelly, Ronald Bremner, Jane Hartley, and Diana Flynn.
© 2014 John Wiley & Sons, Ltd. Published 2014 by John Wiley & Sons, Ltd.

Investigations

- Blood bilirubin and alkaline phosphatase will be elevated
- Gamma-glutamyl transpeptidase (GGT) may be low in some forms of BRIC, hence aiding the diagnosis
- Autoantibodies, including pANCA, immunoglobulins, CRP, ESR
- DNA: mutation screening for the genes involved in bile salt transport to diagnose BRIC (low GGT – *ATP8B1* and *ABCB11*; high GGT – *ABCB4*)
- Liver biopsy: to identify sclerosing cholangitis and associated autoimmune hepatitis (Figure 24.1). Immunohistochemistry for bile salt transporters may aid the diagnosis of BRIC
- Ultrasound: biliary dilatation in sclerosing cholangitis and complications of liver disease (heterogeneous liver, varices, enlarged spleen)
- Magnetic resonance cholangio pancreatography (MRCP): identify the features of sclerosing cholangitis (beading, dilatation, irregular ducts) (Figure 24.2)

Information: Benign recurrent intrahepatic cholestasis (BRIC)

Presents with sudden onset jaundice, pruritis and fat-soluble vitamin deficiency, often during adolescence; may last for weeks to months. The oral contraceptive pill (OCP) may be a precipitating factor. The disease is caused by mutations in *ATP8B1*, *ABCB11* or *ABCB4* , but a precipitating event (such as the OCP) is needed to make it manifest.

Management
- Ursodeoxycholic acid (10–20 mg/kg) and fat-soluble vitamins
- Antipruritics
- If severe, nasobiliary drainage through the nose into the ampulla of Vater reduces the enterohepatic circulation of bile acids and produces relief
- Advice should be given to avoid oestrogen-containing contraception
- Increased oestrogen during the last trimester of pregnancy may cause intrahepatic cholestasis of pregnancy and requires early delivery of the infant

---

Management

- Exclude non-liver causes, e.g. eczema, allergy, scabies
- Avoid soap and keep the skin moisturised, the nails short and cover any bare skin
- Ursodeoxycholic acid 15–30 mg/kg/day

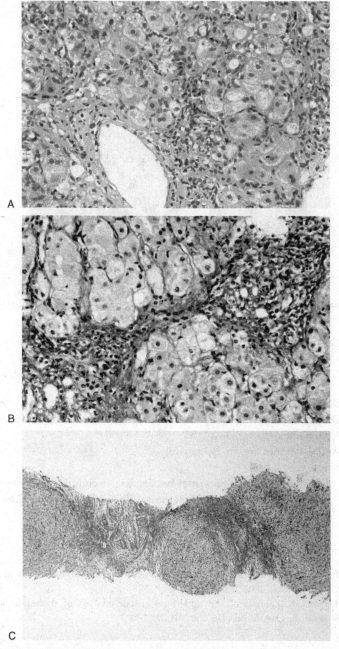

Figure 24.1 (A–C) Histology of chronic hepatitis shows portal inflammation with lymphocytes and plasma cells, hepatocyte balloon degeneration and necrosis, which may be focal (A), or bridging portal tracts with fibrosis (B) or cirrhosis (C), where fibrous tissue links portal tracts and causes nodules.

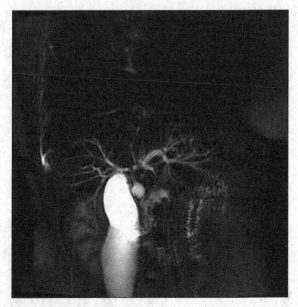

Figure 24.2 Multiple strictures in the biliary tract is demonstrated by magnetic resonance cholangiopancreatography.

- Cholestyramine
  - Under 6 years: 2g (½ sachet)/day
  - Over 6 years: 4g (one sachet)/day
- Rifampicin 3–10 mg/kg once a day
- Ondansteron 2–4 mg bd up to 12 years of age, then 4–8 mg 12–18 years
- Naltrexone 6–20 mg/day
- Antihistamines are rarely effective
- Surgery:
  - External biliary diversion may be beneficial in children with progressive familial intrahepatic cholestasis (PFIC) and Alagille syndrome
  - Intractable pruritis is an indication for liver transplantation

Further reading

Kelly DA. *Diseases of the Liver and Biliary System in Children*, 3rd edn. Oxford: Wiley-Blackwell, 2008, Chapters 3, 4 and 15

Müllenbach R, Lammert F. An update on genetic analysis of cholestatic liver diseases: digging deeper. *Dig Dis* 2011;29:72–77

Key web links

http://www.childliverdisease.org/content/581/Pruritis
http://www.easl.eu/assets/application/files/b664961b2692dc2_file.pdf

Chronic liver disease: ascites

Ascites is the accumulation of fluid in the peritoneal cavity. In liver disease it is secondary to a combination of increased portal vascular hydrostatic pressure and low albumin. It is perpetuated by increased aldosterone and renin production stimulated by reduced intravascular fluid and renal perfusion, hence resulting in renal fluid retention and hyponatraemia.

Important features from history

- There is usually a history of liver disease
- Thrombotic tendency: may indicate Budd–Chiari
- Bone marrow transplantation: may indicate veno-occlusive disease
- Pyrexia, sepsis and abdominal tenderness: may indicate spontaneous bacterial peritonitis

Differential diagnosis

It is important to distinguish ascites due to liver disease from other causes. This can be achieved by measuring the serum–ascites albumin gradient (SAAG).

A gradient of >1.1 g/L gradient = transudate as there is little albumin in the ascites. Causes of a transudate are:

- Chronic liver disease with portal hypertension
- Heart failure or constrictive pericarditis
- Budd–Chiari (see Chapter 23) or veno-occlusive disease
  A gradient of <1.1 g/L = exudate. Causes of an exudate include:
- Infection including spontaneous bacterial peritonitis
- Pancreatitis
- Protein-losing enteropathy or nephrotic syndrome
- Malignancy

Practical Approach to Paediatric Gastroenterology, Hepatology and Nutrition, First Edition.
Deirdre Kelly, Ronald Bremner, Jane Hartley, and Diana Flynn.
© 2014 John Wiley & Sons, Ltd. Published 2014 by John Wiley & Sons, Ltd.

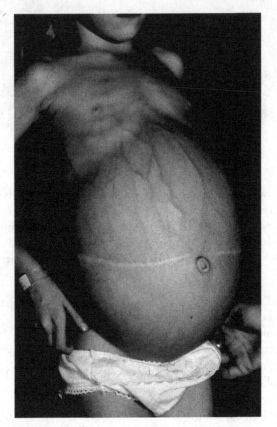

Figure 25.1 Ascites is a common complication of chronic liver disease and presents with abdominal distension and dilated abdominal veins. (Source: Pediatric Gastroenterology and Hepatology, by Deirdre Kelly and Ian Booth, 1997. Reproduced by permission of Elsevier).

Clinical features

The fluid tends to accumulate in the flanks when the child is lying down. It may compromise respiration and enteral intake. In liver disease, palpation of the abdomen is painless. There will be shifting dullness and in massive ascites a fluid thrill can be elicited (Figure 25.1).

Investigations

- FBC: increased white blood cells (WBCs) indicates an infective cause. Platelets and WBCs may be reduced if there is hypersplenism secondary to chronic liver disease
- LFTs: the results will depend on the cause of the liver disease
- U&E: hyponatraemia is often present

- Ascitic tap: this should be carried out with the first presentation of ascites. The ideal place should be determined by ultrasound scan. The tap may be diagnostic (transudate: high SAAG, low LDH, normal glucose, no WBCs with negative Gram stain and no bacteria cultured; exudate: low SAAG, low glucose, high LDH, raised WBCs and bacteria may be identified). Ascitic and serum amylase may identify pancreatitis as the cause of ascites
- Ultrasound scan: identifies the ascites and may also show Budd–Chiari or veno-occlusive disease. Other features of chronic liver disease may be identified

Management

- Spironolactone (1–3 mg/kg/day) is the first-line treatment. Furosemide (0.5–2 mg/kg twice daily) may also be required
- Fluid may need restricting if there is hyponatraemia (therefore feeds should be concentrated to enable adequate calorie intake)
- If there is a low serum albumin concentration, an infusion of 20% HAS (5 ml/kg) over 4 hours with furosemide will increase the oncotic pressure and can be very effective
- Paracentesis to remove the ascites (with venous albumin replacement) is required if there is severe respiratory compromised. There is likely to be rapid re-accumulation
- In refractory cases, metolazone (100–200 μg/kg twice daily), a shunt such as TIPPS or liver transplantation may be indicated

---

Red flags: Bacterial peritonitis

It is important to diagnose spontaneous bacterial peritonitis and therefore tapping the ascites in children who have ascites and pyrexia to gain a sample is essential to guide antibiotic therapy. Therefore, it is better to tap the ascites prior to treatment. The addition of ascites straight into a culture medium bottle provides a better yield of bacteria culture.

Further reading

Giefer MJ, Murray KF, Colletti RB. Pathophysiology, Diagnosis, and Management of Pediatric Ascites. *J Pediatr Gastroenterol Nutr* 2011;52:503–513

Key web link

http://www.naspghan.org/wmspage.cfm?parm1=103

Chronic liver disease: haematemesis or meleana

Gastrointestinal bleeding due to variceal bleeding is common in children with chronic liver disease or extrahepatic portal venous obstruction. This is a medical emergency requiring immediate action and referral to a specialist centre for endoscopy and management.

Differential diagnosis

- Gastric or duodenal ulceration secondary to the use of steroids
- Stress ulceration due to end-stage liver disease

Management

- Cross-match: at least 2 units of packed cells
- Fluid resuscitate with colloid and blood (transfuse to Hb 10 g/mL only)
- Correct coagulopathy and thrombocytopenia
- Fluid: maintain normal glucose, correct electrolyte derangement
- Octreotide (3–5 µg/kg/hour)
- Pass a nasogastric tube and keep on free drainage to identify blood loss
- Nil-by-mouth
- Ranitidine (3 mg/kg three times daily, IV) and oral sucralphate (<2 years – 250 mg four times daily; 2–12 years – 500 mg four times daily; >12 years – 1 g four times daily)
- Blood and urine culture and start broad-spectrum antibiotics, e.g. Tazocin 90 mg/kg tds

Practical Approach to Paediatric Gastroenterology, Hepatology and Nutrition, First Edition.
Deirdre Kelly, Ronald Bremner, Jane Hartley, and Diana Flynn.
© 2014 John Wiley & Sons, Ltd. Published 2014 by John Wiley & Sons, Ltd.

148

- Upper GI endoscopy with variceal band ligation or sclerotherapy to gastric varices; monitor fluid input and output as may develop renal insufficiency
  If bleeding continues, other treatments may include:
- Vasopressin (initial 0.3 units/kg over 30 minutes, then 0.3 units/kg/ hour, increasing up to 1 unit/kg/hour if necessary) or terlipressin (initial 2 mg, then 1–2 mg every 4–6 hours)
- Transjugular intrahepatic portosystemic shunting (only available in specialised centres) may be required to control the bleeding

Further investigations

Ultrasound scan: to identify the portal venous flow. If this is absent or reversed, liver transplantation may be indicated.

Key web link

http://www.aasld.org/practiceguidelines/Documents/Bookmarked%
20Practice%20Guidelines/Prevention%20and%20Management%20
of%20Gastro%20Varices%20and%20Hemorrhage.pdf

Children with incidental abnormal liver biochemistry

Hepatic transaminases (AST/ALT) may be increased due to primary liver disease or the first presentation of a multisystem disease (Table 27.1).

Conditions that commonly present in this way include:

- Non-alcoholic fatty liver disease (NAFLD)
- Non-alcoholic steatoheaptitis (NASH) (see Nutrition section):
- Sclerosing cholangitis
- Alpha-1-antitrypsin deficiency
- Wilson's disease

Important features of history

- Central obesity
- Hypertension
- Family history of liver disease or emphysema
- Change in bowel habit, abdominal pain or blood in stool

Practical Approach to Paediatric Gastroenterology, Hepatology and Nutrition, First Edition.
Deirdre Kelly, Ronald Bremner, Jane Hartley, and Diana Flynn.
© 2014 John Wiley & Sons, Ltd. Published 2014 by John Wiley & Sons, Ltd.

Table 27.1 Specific investigations for abnormal transaminases

Condition	Investigations	Management
Alpha-1-antitrypsin deficiency	See Chapter 17	See Chapter 17
Sclerosing cholangitis	See Chapter 25	See Chapter 25
Wilson's disease	See Chapter 22	See Chapter 22
Non-alcoholic fatty liver disease	Bloods: metabolic syndrome (elevated triglycerides, reduced HDL cholesterol, raised fasting plasma glucose) Ultrasound: hyperreflective due to the brightness of fat in the liver Liver biopsy: fatty infiltration, hepatitis, fibrosis	Weight loss and exercise (no benefit from ursodeoxycholic acid, vitamin E)

HDL, high density lipoprotein.

Further reading

Chalasani N, Younossi Z, Lavine JE, *et al*. The diagnosis and management of non-alcoholic fatty liver disease: Practice Guideline by the American Association for the Study of Liver Diseases, American College of Gastroenterology, and the American Gastroenterological Association. *Hepatology* 2012;55:2005–2023

Key web link

http://www.naspghan.org/user-assets/Documents/pdf/CDHNF%20Old%20Site/Nutrition%20and%20Obesity%20MPR/Medical%20Professional%20Summary%20Statement%20on%20NAFLD.pdf

The child with cystic fibrosis

Cystic fibrosis (CF) is the most common life-limiting autosomal recessive disorder of Caucasians. The defect in the cystic fibrosis transmembrane regulator (CFTR) protein causes an inability to maintain normal hydration of luminal tracts, which leads to thickened secretions and obstruction. As survival with lung disease improves, the recognition of liver and bowel disease is increasing.

Gastrointestinal manifestations of cystic fibrosis include:
- Meconium ileus
- Distal intestinal obstruction
- Rectal prolapse
- Liver steatosis
- Focal or multilobular biliary cirrhosis
- Portal hypertension
- Cholelithiasis
- Pancreatic insufficiency due to chronic or recurrent pancreatitis

Gastrointestinal disease

- Meconium ileus
- Distal intestinal obstruction syndrome

Hepatobiliary disease

Liver disease develops in a third of CF patients and causes 2.5% of CF deaths (Figure 28.1). It is more common in male CF patients and those with meconium ileus as a neonate.

Practical Approach to Paediatric Gastroenterology, Hepatology and Nutrition, First Edition.
Deirdre Kelly, Ronald Bremner, Jane Hartley, and Diana Flynn.
© 2014 John Wiley & Sons, Ltd. Published 2014 by John Wiley & Sons, Ltd.

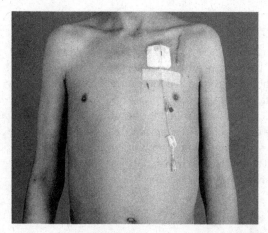

Figure 28.1 Liver disease in cystic fibrosis may present with gradual onset of abdominal distension, malnutrition and bruising secondary to portal hypertension.

In the neonate it may cause prolonged jaundice (which resolves), neonatal hepatitis, fat-soluble vitamin deficiency (especially vitamin K), or inspissated bile syndrome. In older children it presents with hepatomegaly and abnormal transaminases and may remain subclinical until advanced.

Portal hypertension with hypersplenism and variceal bleeding occurs with the development of cirrhosis. Liver function may be maintained for years prior to decompensation.

Investigations

- Ultrasound scan will identify cirrhosis, splenomegaly and steatosis
- Liver biopsy is required if there is doubt about the diagnosis or to stage the disease. Typical histological findings are steatosis, varying degrees of fibrosis, inspissated bile and dilated bile ducts, and, rarely, bile duct proliferation
- Follow-up Debray et al, 2011: monitor with:
  - Liver biochemistry and ultrasound to detect the development of liver disease
  - Alpha-fetoprotein to detect the possible development of hepatocellular carcinoma
  - Upper gastrointestinal endoscopy to detect the development of varices in those with cirrhosis

Management

- Ursodeoxycholic acid (20 mg/kg/day) is used to improve bile flow
- Variceal bleeding requires treatment (see Chapter 26)
- TIPSS should be considered for recurrent bleeding when liver function is maintained
- Liver transplant is indicated for hepatic decompensation, ascites and jaundice or intractable variceal bleeding, which needs to be carried out prior to significant deterioration of lung function (FEV_1 < 50%). Lung function stabilises post transplant
- Nutrition: see Nutrition section

Further reading

Debray D, Kelly D, Houwen R, Strandvik B, Colombo C. Best practice guidance for the diagnosis and management of cystic fibrosis-associated liver disease. *J Cyst Fibros* 2011;10(Suppl 2):S29–36

The child with liver disease following chemotherapy

CHAPTER 29

Up to 30% of children develop liver complications during chemotherapy.

Differential diagnosis

- Infection: any infection; Candida and cytomegalovirus are common
- Graft-versus-host disease (GvHD): acute (7–50 days) or chronic (>100 days)
- Veno-occlusive disease (VOD): more likely with busulphan/ radiotherapy
- Drug toxicity:
  - Actinomycin: hepatitis (may be severe leading to liver synthetic dysfunction)
  - Methotrexate: steatosis and fibrosis
  - Mercaptopurine (6-MCP): hepatic necrosis and fibrosis
  - Doxorubicin: hepatitis

History and examination

- Drug history
- Skin rash and diarrhea may develop in acute GvHD
- Stools may be pale in chronic GvHD due to loss of bile ducts
- Liver is enlarged and tender, abdominal distension due to ascites, raised jugular venous pressure and large weight gain with VOD
- Infection with fever

See table 29.1 for investigations

Practical Approach to Paediatric Gastroenterology, Hepatology and Nutrition, First Edition.
Deirdre Kelly, Ronald Bremner, Jane Hartley, and Diana Flynn.
© 2014 John Wiley & Sons, Ltd. Published 2014 by John Wiley & Sons, Ltd.

Table 29.1 Specific investigations for hepatic complications of chemotherapy

Complication	Investigation
Infection	Culture: blood, urine, CSF
	PCR for viruses especially CMV
	Chest X-ray
	CT: identify Candida in liver
	Liver or bone marrow biopsy for culture
VOD	Ultrasound: shows retrograde portal venous flow and increased hepatic resistance
	CT angiogram: may identify poor flow in the hepatic veins
GvHD	Skin biopsy
	Liver biopsy: vanishing bile ducts
Drug-induced liver disease	History of drugs used
	Liver biopsy

CMV, cytomegalovirus; CSF, cerebrospinal fluid; PCR, polymerase chain reaction.

Management

- Infection:
  - Dependent on the causative organism
  - Ambisone and ganciclovir until culture results are known
- GvHD:
  - Increase immunosuppression with steroids/ciclosporin or tacrolimus
  - Liver transplant may be indicated in chronic GvHD
  - Ursodeoxycholic acid may provide relief for pruritis
- VOD:
  - Treatment of cholestasis and ascites
  - Defibrotide is a local thrombolytic which has reduced mortality rate

- Drug-induced liver disease:
  ◦ Discontinue drug
  ◦ Long-term follow-up if fibrosis develops (6-thioguanine leads to non-cirrhotic portal hypertension and is now no longer used)

Key web link

http://onlinelibrary.wiley.com/doi/10.1002/14651858.CD008205
.pub2/pdf

The management of a child with acute liver failure

Management should be at a transplant centre with the aims to be supportive to prevent complications, identify and provide specific treatment, and identify those children who require super urgent liver transplant. Medications are listed in Table 30.1.

- No sedation as it masks encephalopathy
- Minimal handling
- Consider central venous access
- Regular monitoring:
  - Continuous cutaneous oximetry and ECG monitor
  - Core–toe temperature
  - Neurological observations, baseline EEG
  - Gastric pH (>5.0)
  - Urine output maintain 0.5–2ml/kg/hour
  - Blood glucose/BM monitoring (>4mmol/L)
  - Acid–base balance, lactate
  - Electrolytes (including magnesium, calcium and phosphate), ammonia
  - Alkaline phosphatase, AST, ALT, GGT, serum bilirubin, albumin
  - Coagulation screen
  - Plasma and urine osmolality
- Fluid management:
  - Fluid balance 50–75% maintenance
  - Dextrose infusions to maintain BM (10–50% glucose required)
  - Maintain circulating volume with colloid (4.5% or 20% human albumin solution)
  - Maintain normal electrolytes and acid base

Practical Approach to Paediatric Gastroenterology, Hepatology and Nutrition, First Edition.
Deirdre Kelly, Ronald Bremner, Jane Hartley, and Diana Flynn.
© 2014 John Wiley & Sons, Ltd. Published 2014 by John Wiley & Sons, Ltd.

Table 30.1 Medication used in acute liver failure

Drug	Dose
Vitamin K	<1 year 2.5 mg/dose od IV
	>1 year 5 mg/dose od IV
	>10 year 10 mg/dose od IV
Antacids	Ranitidine 1–3 mg/kg/dose tds IV
	or
	Omeprazole 0.5 mg/kg/dose bd IV or orally
	Sucralphate 250–500 mg/dose qds (if gastric pH remains <5)
Lactulose	2–4 ml/kg/dose tds
N-acetylcysteine	150 mg/kg/day continuous infusion (only if paracetamol overdose)
Broad-spectrum antibiotics:	
Tazocin	90 mg/kg/dose tds
Metronidazole	8 mg/kg/dose tds IV (bd for neonates up to 1 month)
Antifungals:	3–6 mg/kg/day IV
Fluconazole	Neonate under 2 weeks: 3–6 mg/kg on first day, then 3 mg/kg every 72 hours
or	Neonate 2–4 weeks: 3–6 mg/kg on first day, then 3 mg/kg every 48 hours
L-Amphotericin (Ambisome)	3 mg/kg/day IV
Antiviral treatment:	
Aciclovir	<3 months: 10 mg/kg tds IV
Must be started in all infants	3 months–12 years: 250 mg/m^2 tds IV
	>12 years: 5 mg/kg tds IV
	NB: Double the dose in immunocompromised or severe illness

- Nutrition:
  - Nil orally until galactosaemia, tyrosinaemia, urea cycle disorder ruled out
  - Consider parenteral nutrition (PN) if unable to feed
- Coagulation should not be supported unless discussed with the transplant centre

Prognosis

ALF secondary to hepatitis A, autoimmune hepatitis and paracetamol toxicity are most likely to recover with appropriate treatment.

See Chapter 31 for indications for transplantation in acute liver failure.

Children with grade III encephalopathy should be referred to intensive care. If children require an anaesthetic (such as for central line insertion), they may need PICU admission.

Complications

Hypoglycaemia

Severe hypoglycaemia (blood glucose <3.5 mmol/L) contributes to neurological impairment and other organ dysfunction. Refractory hypoglycaemia carries a poor prognostic implication.

Management
- Intravenous glucose administration (10–50% dextrose)
- Avoid hyperglycaemia

Coagulopathy and bleeding

Prothrombin time is the most sensitive measure of hepatic synthesis and determines need for transplantation. Disseminated intravascular coagulation may develop in sepsis.

Management
- Daily dose of IV vitamin K
- Do not routinely correct coagulopathy with blood products, e.g. fresh frozen plasma (FFP) or cryoprecipitate, as PT is a sensitive guide to prognosis and need for liver transplantation
- Once the decision to list for transplant has been made, start correcting PT >40 seconds (to avoid risk of bleeding)
- Use FFP (10–15 ml/kg every 6 hours), cryoprecipitate and platelets (if required)
- Consider use of recombinant factor VIIa (rFVIIa) for refractory bleeding
- Haemofiltration may be required to control fluid balance

Encephalopathy

The grade of encephalopathy, clinical features and management strategy are listed in Table 30.2.

- Brain death associated with cerebral oedema is the commonest cause of death
- May be exacerbated by sepsis, GI bleeding and electrolyte disturbances
- Children may fluctuate rapidly from one grade to another
- Suspected raised intracranial pressure alone is *not* an indication for a cranial CT unless there are unilateral neurological signs (indicating intracranial bleed)

Convulsions

- Clinical presentation may be atypical or occult in children
- May be caused by underlying cause of acute liver failure (toxic injury, viral, metabolic, etc.), electrolyte imbalance, cerebral oedema

Management

- Consider mannitol infusion if caused by possible cerebral oedema and plasma sodium <135 mmol/L: 0.5–2 g/kg over 1 hour (2.5–10 ml/kg of 20% mannitol)
- Repeat every 6–8 hours for a maximum of 48 hours
- Measure osmolarity every 12 hours (max 310 mOsmol/kg)

Renal dysfunction

- Defined as urine output <0.5 mL/kg/hour in 2 consecutive hours
- Possible causes: hepatorenal syndrome, dehydration, low central venous pressure (CVP)/cardiac output

Management

- Colloid challenge: 10–20 ml/kg over 30–60 minutes; repeat if no response
- If CVP is high (>8 mmHg): start renal dose of dopamine 2–5 µg/kg/min
- If no response: start furosemide – 1–2 mg/kg stat IV
- If established renal failure:
  - Furosemide infusion: 0.25–1 mg/kg/hour
  - Haemofiltration

Metabolic acidosis

- Consider following causes: hypovolaemia, hypoxia, sepsis, renal failure

Table 30.2 Encephalopathy grade and management

Grade	EEG changes	Clinical manifestations	Management
I	Minimal	Mild intellectual impairment, irritable, lethargy/mildly obtunded, disturbed sleep–awake cycle	Head elevated at 20°, no neck flexion Review fluid balance; may require haemofiltration to maintain neutral balance
II	Generalised slowing of rhythm	Drowsiness, confusion, inappropriate/odd behaviour, disorientation/not recognising parents, mood swings, photophobia	All children who develop grade II encephalopathy should be discussed with ITU
III (stupor)	Grossly abnormal slowing	Unresponsive to verbal commands, markedly confused, aggressive, delirious, hyperreflexia, positive Babinski sign	Admit to ITU for elective ventilation CT-scan: consider if *focal* cerebral lesion, i.e. bleeding, suspected only Give mannitol: 0.5–2 g/kg over 1 hour (2.5–10 ml/kg of 20% mannitol) Repeat every 6–8 hours for a maximum of 48 hours Measure osmolarity every 12 hours (max 310 mOsmol/kg) May need to consider thiopentone: 4–8 mg/kg stat IV

Table 30.2 (*Continued*)

Grade	EEG changes	Clinical manifestations	Management
IV (coma)	Delta waves, decreased amplitudes	Unconscious, initial response to pain present, later decerebrate or decorticate response to pain present or absent, areflexia	0.5–3 mg/kg/hour infusion

Management
- Treat if base excess (BE) >10 and pH <7.25
- 8.4% sodium bicarbonate IV as follows:

$$\text{ml bicarbonate} = \frac{\text{weight (kg)} \times \text{base deficit}}{6} \text{ (i.e. half correct)}$$

Sepsis
Signs of sepsis may be subtle, e.g. rise in heart rate or core–toe temperature gradient, fall in blood pressure or urine output, hypo- or hyperglycaemia, hypothermia, deterioration in mental state, fits, increasing acidosis.

Management
- Septic screen, omitting lumbar puncture and supra-pubic puncture
- Start broad spectrum antibiotics and antifungals 'blind' (as per baseline drugs) and escalate after discussion with microbiologist

Indications for liver transplant

CHAPTER 31

Chronic liver disease

Causes
- Graft versus host disease
- Budd chiari
- hepatopulmonary or portopulmonary syndrome
- Biliary atresia
- Alpha-1-antitrypsin deficiency
- Autoimmune hepatitis type I and II
- Sclerosing cholangitis
- Wilson's disease
- Cystic fibrosis liver disease
- Progressive familial intrahepatic cholestasis (all types)
- Alagille syndrome
- Glycogen storage diseases type 3 and 4
- Tyrosinaemia type 1
- Fibrocystic disease with Caroli syndrome and renal failure

Indications
- Irreversible liver decompensation
- Severe portal hypertension: unresponsive to therapy
- Growth failure or developmental delay due to liver disease
- Unacceptable quality of life
- Life expectancy <18 months

Acute liver failure

This is a multisystem disorder in which severe acute impairment of liver function with or without encephalopathy occurs with no recognised underlying chronic liver disease.

Practical Approach to Paediatric Gastroenterology, Hepatology and Nutrition, First Edition.
Deirdre Kelly, Ronald Bremner, Jane Hartley, and Diana Flynn.
© 2014 John Wiley & Sons, Ltd. Published 2014 by John Wiley & Sons, Ltd.

Common causes
- Viral hepatitis A,B,E, seronegative
- Autoimmune hepatitis I or II
- Wilson's disease
- Paracetamol poisoning

Indications
- Acute liver failure in children less than 2 years old with INR >4 or Grade 3/4 encephalopathy
- Acute liver failure due to seronegative hepatitis, hepatitis A, or hepatitis B or an idiosyncratic drug reaction
  - Any grade of encephalopathy, and any three from the following:
  - Unfavourable aetiology (idiosyncratic drug reaction, seronegative hepatitis)
  - Age <10 years
  - Jaundice to encephalopathy time >7 days
  - Serum bilirubin >300 µmol/l
  - Prothrombin time >50 seconds
  - INR >3.5
- Acute liver failure due to Wilson's disease, Budd-Chiari syndrome, paracetamol poisoning or early graft dysfunction
  - As per the indication for adults

Liver tumours

Indications
- Unresectable hepatoblastoma (without active extrahepatic disease)
- Unresectable benign liver tumours with disabling symptoms

Metabolic liver disease with extrahepatic disease

Indications
- Crigler Najjar syndrome
- Urea cycle defects
- Hypercholesterolaemia
- Organic acidaemias
- Primary hyperoxaluria

Complications following liver transplant

CHAPTER 32

Complications may occur any time post transplant:
- Surgical complications: hepatic artery thrombosis, bile duct leak (<14 days)
- Graft rejection: acute (7–10 days) and chronic (at any time)
- Infection
- Post-transplant lymphoproliferative disease (PTLD)
- Relapse of disease: autoimmune hepatitis or sclerosing cholangitis
- Development of *de novo* post-transplant hepatitis (at any time)

It is important to keep in contact with the transplant centre to discuss problems post transplant.

Investigation (Algorithm 32.1)

- LFTs: AST and ALT will be raised with all complications; GGT, alkaline phosphatase and bilirubin may be raised if there is bile duct involvement/obstruction
- PT: to assess graft function
- Albumin: may be low in graft dysfunction or PTLD
- FBC: anaemia is common in PTLD
- PCR: Epstein–Barr virus (EBV) and cytomegalovirus (CMV) PCR and serology will identify acute infection
- Autoantibodies: relapse of autoimmune hepatitis or the development of *de novo* hepatitis
- Immunoglobulins: will be raised with relapsed autoimmune hepatitis
- Ultrasound scan: to assess vascular or biliary causes

Practical Approach to Paediatric Gastroenterology, Hepatology and Nutrition, First Edition.
Deirdre Kelly, Ronald Bremner, Jane Hartley, and Diana Flynn.
© 2014 John Wiley & Sons, Ltd. Published 2014 by John Wiley & Sons, Ltd.

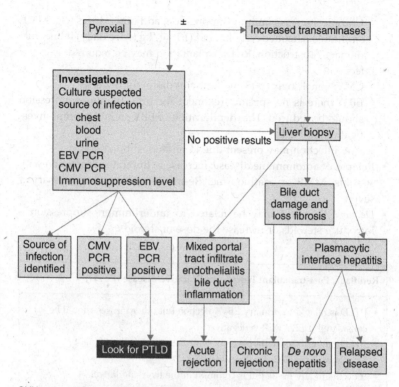

CMV, cytomegalovirus; EBV, Epstein–Barr virus; PCR, polymerase chain reaction; PTLD, post-transplant lymphoproliferative disease.

Algorithm 32.1 Investigations post liver transplant

- Liver biopsy:
  - Acute rejection: endothelitis and inflammation
  - Chronic rejection: bile duct damage
  - Viral inclusions in CMV, EBER stain positive if EBV infection, interface hepatitis with plasma cells in relapsed autoimmune hepatitis or post-transplant *de novo* hepatitis

Management

- Rejection:
  - Acute: pulsed methyl prednisolone 10 mg/kg/day IV for 3 days with ranitidine. Maintenance immunosuppression should be increased or other agents added [mycophenolate mofitil (MMF) (10–20 mg/kg twice daily)]

- ○ Chronic: Increase immunosuppression, add other drugs (e.g. MMF, sirolimus). Ursodeoxycholic acid (10 mg/kg twice daily) if bile duct damage/obstruction. Re-transplantation may be required
- Infection:
  - ○ CMV: ganciclovir IV (5 mg/kg twice daily) for 3 weeks
  - ○ EBV: there is no specific treatment for EBV. Immunosuppression should be reduced. The identification of EBV should prompt investigation of PTLD
  - ○ Any infection may present due to immunosuppression
- Relapse of autoimmune disease: increase in immunosuppression with steroids, MMF or azathioprine. Re-transplant may be necessary if severe
- *De novo* hepatitis: may be related to under-immunosuppression – introduce steroids or increase the dose of steroids

---

Red flags: Post-transplant lymphoproliferative disease (PTLD)

- PTLD is related to primary EBV infection but other viruses should be considered if EBV PCR is negative
- PTLD ranges from hyperplasia of lymphatic tissue to malignant lymphoma with B or T cell proliferation
- It occurs in any tissue but is common in the liver and bowel

Investigations:
- Liver, small bowel biopsy
- Chest X-ray and abdominal ultrasound/CT scan to identify lymphadenopathy
- Lymph node histology

Management
- Reduce or stop immunosuppression
- Commence ganciclovir 10 mg/kg/day IV
- For B-cell PTLD:
  - ○ Rituximab once weekly for 4 weeks and monthly immunoglobulins for 1 year
  - ○ Chemotherapy if no response to rituximab or for T-cell PTLD (rare)

Further reading

Evans HM, Kelly DA, McKiernan PJ, Hubscher S. Progressive histological damage in liver allografts following pediatric liver transplantation. *Hepatology* 2006; 43:1109–1117

Key web links

http://www.naspghan.org/user-assets/Documents/pdf/WG%20
Reports%202008/liver%20transplant.pdf

http://www.organdonation.nhs.uk:8001/ukt/about_transplants/organ
_allocation/pdf/paed_protocols_guidelines.pdf

https://www.aasld.org/practiceguidelines/Documents/LongTerm
ManagmentofSuccessfulLT.pdf

Nutrition

Good nutrition is essential for all children, and is often a significant issue for children with chronic diseases. It is essential to recognize when nutrition is compromised before significant growth and developmental effects are seen. For those children with complex nutritional needs specialist support in the form of a multidisciplinary nutritional support team is usually necessary. This sections outlines current methods of nutritional monitoring, gives an overview of common nutritional problems and outlines management strategies for artificial nutrition support where food intake is poor or energy expenditure increased.

Practical Approach to Paediatric Gastroenterology, Hepatology and Nutrition, First Edition.
Deirdre Kelly, Ronald Bremner, Jane Hartley, and Diana Flynn.
© 2014 John Wiley & Sons, Ltd. Published 2014 by John Wiley & Sons, Ltd.

Nutritional monitoring

Growth charts are the best method of monitoring adequate nutritional intake in children. Height and weight should be plotted in all children at each hospital attendance, and during prolonged hospital stays. Serial measurements are important in determining growth patterns. Mid-parental heights and bone age can assist. Note that specialised growth charts are available for several genetic disorders, e.g. trisomy 21. Managing malnutrition is important as it affects duration of hospital stay and increases infection risk.

Red flags: Poor head growth in malnutrition of infancy

In malnutrition there is relative sparing of the brain, therefore poor head growth in this context can indicate severe deficiency. Note that it can also be seen in other conditions, including developmental delay and genetic disorders.

Information: Anthropometry

- Height and weight: at outpatient visits; on admission to hospital; repeat weight weekly and height monthly for inpatients
- Head circumference: in children under 2 years old.
- Additional measurements, e.g. mid-arm circumference for muscle stores, and skinfold thickness (traditionally triceps, scapula) for fat stores

Body mass index (BMI) = weight (kg)/[height (m)]^2

(Continued)

Practical Approach to Paediatric Gastroenterology, Hepatology and Nutrition, First Edition.
Deirdre Kelly, Ronald Bremner, Jane Hartley, and Diana Flynn.
© 2014 John Wiley & Sons, Ltd. Published 2014 by John Wiley & Sons, Ltd.

BMI needs to be plotted on centile charts for meaningful paediatric interpretation as it changes with age and sex. It is useful for both the underweight and obese.

More detailed measures of body composition are available but are usually reserved for research purposes.

Calculation or measurement of energy expenditure and nutritional requirements are sometimes used in certain situations, e.g. paediatric intensive care unit (PICU).

Nutritional screening

A simple scoring system, performed by nurses on hospital admission and intermittently throughout hospital stay in some hospitals, including anthropometry, to alert clinical teams and dietitians to malnutrition risk.

Information: The multidisciplinary nutrition support team

Those with complex nutritional disorders or intestinal failure should be referred to and managed by the local multidisciplinary nutrition support team where available.

Members of the team may include:
- Consultant: usually a gastroenterologist
- Dietitian
- Nutrition nurse specialist
- Pharmacist
- Psychologist
- Speech and language therapist
- Paediatric surgeon
- Microbiologist
- Biochemist

In addition there may be links with a paediatric neurologist, adult gastroenterologist, nutrition support team and/or paediatric liver and small bowel transplant centre.

Further reading

Gerasimidis K, Keane O, Macleod I *et al*. A four-stage evaluation of the Paediatric Yorkhill Malnutrition Score in a tertiary paediatric hospital and a district general hospital. *Br J Nutr* 2010;104:751–756

Hall DM, Cole TJ. What use is the BMI? *Arch Dis Child* 2006;91:283–286

Key web links

http://www.rcpch.ac.uk/growthcharts

MCN consultation: expert paper – growth monitoring: http://www.nice
.org.uk/guidance/index.jsp?action=download&r=true&o=34693

Organisation of nutrition support teams: http://www.bapen.org.uk/
ofnsh/page7.html

Nutrition in the normal infant: breast-feeding

Breast milk provides the optimal nutrition for babies (Table 34.1). Encouragement and support of breast-feeding mothers is important for effective breast-feeding, and breast-feeding advisors and midwives are key in this. Problems need prompt identification and management (Table 34.2). All maternity units are encouraged to be accredited by the UNICEF baby-friendly initiative that supports the mother–baby bond, including standards for optimal support of breast-feeding mothers.

Red flags: Signs of failed breast-feeding

- Failure of breast-feeding due to inadequate milk production is rare
- Dry nappies, weight loss and irritability are signs of dehydration

---

Feeding routines and behaviour

Conflicting advice in popular books and the media is common. Many mothers find that their baby will develop a routine over the first few weeks, with feeding on demand.

Growth

Use new WHO growth charts for all children born after 2009. All babies should be weighed at birth, 5 days and 10 days old. Most babies lose some weight in the first few days of life but this is usually regained by 2 weeks of age. Only 3–7% of babies lose >10% of their birth weight.

Practical Approach to Paediatric Gastroenterology, Hepatology and Nutrition, First Edition.
Deirdre Kelly, Ronald Bremner, Jane Hartley, and Diana Flynn.
© 2014 John Wiley & Sons, Ltd. Published 2014 by John Wiley & Sons, Ltd.

Table 34.1 Benefits of breastfeeding

Benefit to baby	Benefit to mother
Decreased risk of diarrhoeal illness	Decreased risk of breast cancer
Fewer respiratory infections	Decreased risk of type 2 diabetes mellitus later in life
Decreased sudden infant death (SID) risk	Decreased obesity
Improved cognitive function	Cheaper and ready availability
Improved bone mass at 17 years	
Appetite regulation and decreased risk of obesity	
Decreased risk of necrotising enterocolitis in premature babies	

Note that benefits are greater when breast-feeding is exclusive.

Table 34.2 Differential diagnosis of breast-feeding problems

Diagnosis	History	Management
Poor positioning	Bleeding, cracked nipples	Reposition promptly if not latched on properly
	Baby unsettled	Purified lanolin to cracked nipples to prevent scabs (see referenced video)
Candida infection	Painful, very pink nipples	Mother: clotrimazole/ miconazole cream
	Sharp breast pains	Baby: oral nystatin

(Continued)

Table 34.2 (*Continued*)

Diagnosis	History	Management
Blocked duct	Painful area of breast	Frequent breast-feeding
		Apply warm pad to breast prior to feed to aid duct drainage
		Massage towards nipple during feed
		NB: prompt action may prevent mastitis
Mastitis	As for blocked duct with tender, hot red swelling, flu-like symptoms	Feed using the tender breast first
		Hand express between feeds if breasts full
	Fever	Bed rest, back massage ± paracetamol
		If symptoms persist consider antibiotics (see referenced video)
Cow's milk protein intolerance (see Chapter 12)	History of atopy	Trial of cow's milk-free diet for mother
	Baby with irritability, vomiting, diarrhoea or blood in stool, ± eczema	Consider hydrolysed or amino-acid feed

Information: Vitamins in pregnancy and infancy

- Vitamin D: recommended for all mothers during pregnancy and lactation, and infants from 6 months of age or sooner if high risk.
- Vitamin K: deficiency causes bleeding and rarely intracranial haemorrhage. As breast milk is low in vitamin K, babies receive at least three doses of oral vitamin K according to local policy or IM at birth

Further reading

Fisk CM, Crozier SR, Inskip HM *et al*. Breastfeeding and reported morbidity during infancy: findings from the Southampton Women's Survey. *Matern Child Nutr* 2011;7:61–70

Key web links

Healthy child e-learning programme (RCPCH): http://www.rcpch .ac.uk/hcp

Position statement on breastfeeding RCPCH: http://www.rcpch.ac.uk/ sites/default/files/RCPCH%20Position%20Statement%2020.06.11.pdf

UNICEF baby friendly initiative: http://www.unicef.org.uk/Baby Friendly/Health-Professionals/New-Baby-Friendly-Standards/

Short video clips for correct positioning for breastfeeding: http://www .unicef.org.uk/BabyFriendly/Resources/AudioVideo/What-good -breastfeeding-looks-like/

NHS website pages on breastfeeding: http://www.nhs.uk/Planners/ breastfeeding/Pages/breastfeeding-tips.aspx

Pages from Birth to Five online: http://www.dh.gov.uk/prod_consum _dh/groups/dh_digitalassets/documents/digitalasset/dh_107706.pdf

Nutrition in the normal infant: infant formulae

Mothers who bottle feed should receive the same level of support for feeding as breast-feeding mothers (Table 35.1). The cost of bottle feeding an infant is estimated at £450 for the first year.

General advice and support

- Encourage skin–to-skin contact and eye contact with baby during feeds
- Keep baby upright, teat full of milk to avoid air swallowing
- Current recommendations: demand feed every 2–4 hours
- Normal requirements: once feeding established 150 ml/kg/day for the first few weeks of life (see link)
  Common problems with formula feeding are listed in Table 35.1.

Which milk to choose?

- For an excellent summary see the link 'Infant milks in the UK'
- Avoid soya formula <6 months of age
- Goat's milk formula is not suitable for babies <1 year

Information: Current WHO recommendations for making up formula

---

Use water at least 70 °C to decrease contamination risk by *Salmonella* or *Cronobacter sakazakii*. These are uncommon but can be serious, and mortality has historically been high.

Practical Approach to Paediatric Gastroenterology, Hepatology and Nutrition, First Edition. Deirdre Kelly, Ronald Bremner, Jane Hartley, and Diana Flynn.
© 2014 John Wiley & Sons, Ltd. Published 2014 by John Wiley & Sons, Ltd.

Table 35.1 Common problems with formula feeding

Diagnosis	History	Management
Wind/colic	Unsettled after feed	Encourage winding
		Severe colic may be related to cow's milk protein intolerance (CMPI)
	Air swallowing	
	Crying	1-week trial of hydrolysed formula
		Exclude UTI if excessive crying
		Probiotics may help
Cow's milk protein intolerance (see Chapter 12)	Vomiting, diarrhoea or blood in stool ± eczema	Change to hydrolysed feed
		If severe consider elemental feed
	Family history of atopy	
Constipation (see Chapter 14)	Infrequent hard stools	Check formula made up correctly (see Information: Current WHO recommendations for making up formulabox)
	Check that meconium passed in first 24–48 hours	
Gastro-oesophageal reflux (see Chapter 3)	Crying, back arching and refusing feeds	See Chapter 3
		Also consider CMPI
Obesity	Weight crosses centiles upwards	Check formula made up correctly
		Discuss feed frequency and hunger signs
	More likely with formula milk than breast-feeding	After 6 weeks old, night feed not usually required
		Medical causes are rare: plot length and orbitofrontal cortex

Further reading

Douglas PS, Hill PS. The crying baby: what approach? *Curr Opin Pediatr* 2011;23:523–529

Hemachandra AH, Howards PP, Furth SL, Klebanoff MA. Birth weight, postnatal growth, and risk for high blood pressure at 7 years of age: results from the Collaborative Perinatal Project. *Pediatrics* 2007;119:e1264–1270

Lempainen J, Tauriainen S, Vaarala O *et al*. Interaction of enterovirus infection and Cow's milk-based formula nutrition in type 1 diabetes-associated autoimmunity. *Diabetes Metab Res Rev* 2012;28:177–185

Singhal A, Kennedy K, Lanigan J *et al*. Nutrition in infancy and long-term risk of obesity: evidence from 2 randomized controlled trials. *Am J Clin Nutr* 2010;92:1133–1144

Key web links

Correct positioning for bottle feeding: http://www.nhs.uk/Conditions/pregnancy-and-baby/Pages/bottle-feeding-advice.aspx

Infant milks in the UK: http://www.cwt.org.uk/pdfs/infantsmilk_web.pdf

http://www.nhs.uk/Planners/birthtofive/Pages/bottle-feeding.aspx

Nutrition in premature infants

Babies born prematurely (<37 weeks' gestation) have different nutritional challenges depending on gestational age at delivery. Those <34 weeks' gestation may not be able to suck from the breast/bottle. Very low birth weight (VLBW) infants (<1500 g) and extremely low birth weight (ELBW) infants (<1000 g) have increased fluid and calorie requirements and have greater risk of necrotising enterocolitis (NEC). Breast milk is the starting feed of choice for all premature infants, with lower NEC rates and better nutrient absorption, and supplies LC-PUFA. Mothers should be involved in feeding plans and supported to express breast milk until infants can suckle (see link). Skin-to-skin contact between baby and mother is encouraged.

Feeding infants <1500g birth weight

Most of these infants will require parenteral nutrition (PN) with gradual introduction of enteral feeding once clinically stable.

- PN is increased over 4–5 days to around 150 mL/kg/day
- Early enteral feeding with expressed breast milk (EBM) is beneficial, but may increase rates of NEC (Table 36.1), so standardised programmes have been introduced in many units, e.g. minimal (trophic) feeds for the first 6–8 days followed by increments of 20 mL/kg/day until target volume/calorie intake is reached
- Breast-milk fortifier is used to achieve adequate calorie density once volumes reach 150 mL/kg/day
- Volumes of up to 180 ml/kg of feeds may be required.
- If EBM cannot be used, then a low osmolarity preterm formula should be used Supplementation of fat-soluble vitamins, calcium, phosphate and iron may be required

Practical Approach to Paediatric Gastroenterology, Hepatology and Nutrition, First Edition.
Deirdre Kelly, Ronald Bremner, Jane Hartley, and Diana Flynn.
© 2014 John Wiley & Sons, Ltd. Published 2014 by John Wiley & Sons, Ltd.

Table 36.1 Factors affecting necrotising enterocolitis risk

Decreased risk	Increased risk
Human milk	Formula milk
Probiotics	Xanthum gum-based thickeners in feed
Lactoferrin	Blood transfusion
	Ranitidine

Encouraging oral feeds

Oromotor development is aided by:

- Non-nutritive sucking
- Stroking cheeks, lips, tongue and gums

Information: Milk banks

- Aim to increase amount of available breast milk primarily for premature infants whose mothers cannot provide their own milk
- Milk is accepted from mothers with babies under 6 months old
- Exclusion criteria for donors: smoking, regular alcohol intake >1–2 units once or twice a week; positive HBV, HCV, HIV 1 or 2, HTLV I or II or syphilis. Current/recent drug users and those at increased risk of CJD are also excluded

Outcome

Improved nutrition in premature infants leads to decreased complications, including NEC, and improves long-term developmental potential, with decreased cerebral palsy risk.

Further reading

McCallie KR, Lee HC, Mayer O, Cohen RS, Hintz SR, Rhine WD. Improved outcomes with a standardized feeding protocol for very low birth weight infants. *J Perinatol* 2011;31 (Suppl 1):S61–67

Stephens BE, Walden RV, Gargus RA *et al*. First-week protein and energy intakes are associated with 18-month developmental outcomes in extremely low birth weight infants. *Pediatrics* 2009;123:1337–1343

Sullivan S, Schanler RJ, Kim JH *et al.* An exclusively human milk-based diet is associated with a lower rate of necrotizing enterocolitis than a diet of human milk and bovine milk-based products. *J Pediatr* 2010;156:562–567.e1

Key web links

UK association for milk banking: http://www.ukamb.org/

NICE guideline on milk banks (July 2011): http://guidance.nice.org.uk/CG93

Expressing breast milk: http://www.nhs.uk/Conditions/pregnancy-and-baby/pages/expressing-storing-breast-milk.aspx

Problems with weaning

WHO recommendations are to encourage exclusive breast-feeding with introduction of solids around the age of 6 months.

Weaning before 16 weeks is not advised due to bowel immaturity. Delayed weaning much beyond 6 months has been linked to coeliac disease, allergy, iron deficiency and aversion to solids.

Important aspects

- Family eating together: encourages good eating patterns and development of social aspects of feeding
- Refusal of lumpy foods: history of tube feeding, late introduction of solids, gastro-oesophageal reflux

---

Information: Starting to wean

- Introduce daily tastes when hungry and not too tired, sitting with good head control and showing interest in food
- Salt should not be added to infant foods due to immature renal system
- Introduce lumps gradually
- Baby-led weaning is where solid foods are given to hold, rather than the baby being spoon fed. This may improve longer-term food intake regulation
- A combination of spoon feeding and baby-led weaning is recommended

---

Practical Approach to Paediatric Gastroenterology, Hepatology and Nutrition, First Edition.
Deirdre Kelly, Ronald Bremner, Jane Hartley, and Diana Flynn.
© 2014 John Wiley & Sons, Ltd. Published 2014 by John Wiley & Sons, Ltd.

Information: Vitamins and minerals in the older infant

Vitamin D supplements should be prescribed for all infants receiving
<500 ml of formula per day and children aged 1–5 years.

Further reading

Fewtrell MS. The evidence for public health recommendations on infant feeding.
Early Hum Dev 2011;87:715–721

Key web links

http://www.nhs.uk/Planners/birthtofive/Pages/Weaningfirststeps
.aspx

For the e-version of the *Birth to Five* (2009) chapters on weaning see:
http://www.dh.gov.uk/prod_consum_dh/groups/dh_digitalassets/
documents/digitalasset/dh_107710.pdf

The infant or child with poor feeding

Poor feeding can be due many factors, including poor coordination of suck/swallow, gastrointestinal disease or social factors. Investigation is required where there is weight loss or inadequate weight gain, choking on feeds or recurrent aspiration pneumonia (Table 38.1). Management depends on the underlying cause.

Important features from history

- Delay in establishing feeds: may indicate an underlying neurological condition
- Change in feed tolerance with change of feed, e.g. breast to formula or on weaning – consider food allergy
- Early illness or prematurity
- Children/adolescents with autistic spectrum disorders may have a very limited food repertoire, only eating a very few selected foods. Some children with Asperger's report little appetite and no hunger and consequently may eat little.

Information: Weight faltering

- Poor suck or poor appetite by 6 weeks of age, with maternal re-enforcement, are predictors of non-organic weight faltering in infants, with subtle oromotor delay
- Weight faltering before 8 weeks of age is associated with decreased IQ at age 8 years
- Maternal and socioeconomic factors are *not* usually significant, but postnatal depression, older maternal age and Asian families have been associated

---

Practical Approach to Paediatric Gastroenterology, Hepatology and Nutrition, First Edition.
Deirdre Kelly, Ronald Bremner, Jane Hartley, and Diana Flynn.
© 2014 John Wiley & Sons, Ltd. Published 2014 by John Wiley & Sons, Ltd.

Table 38.1 Differential diagnosis of poor feeding in infancy

Diagnosis	History	Investigation	Management
Delayed/ abnormal oromotor development	Choking on feeds, drooling, recurrent aspiration, prematurity, hypotonia	Speech and language therapist (SALT) assessment with videofluoroscopy	Oral stimulation programme (SALT)
			Thickened feeds
		Exclude neurodevelopmental disorder	Enteral feeding if unsafe swallow
Cleft lip/ palate		ENT referral	Specially designed teats
			Corrective surgery
Congenital heart disease	Sweating with feeds, shortness of breath, central cyanosis	Echocardiography and cardiology review	Smaller more frequent feeds
			Consider enteral feeding
Foregut dysmotility	Vomiting	Barium meal	Jejunal feeding

(Continued)

Table 38.1 (*Continued*)

Diagnosis	History	Investigation	Management
Tongue-tie	Difficulties in breast-feeding have been reported		Consider ligation if severe
Pyloric stenosis	Projectile vomiting	See Chapter 3	Pyloromyotomy
Reflux oesophagitis	Recurrent vomiting, arching of the back poor sleeping, crying	See Chapter 3	See Chapter 3
Cow's milk protein intolerance	Vomiting and crying, eczema, family history of atopy or allergy	See Chapter 12	See Chapter 12
Tracheo-oesophageal fistula	Choking, drooling, coughing and/or cyanosis on feeding with aspiration, poor feeding, history of polyhydramnios	Exclude trisomy 21 or 18, CHARGE, VACTERL Attempt to pass NG tube into stomach; X-ray	Surgical: classed as a surgical emergency

Causes of poor feeding in the older child

- Consider underlying gastrointestinal disease, pain, neglect, autistic spectrum, eating disorders, cachexia
- Children with food neophobia eat only a very limited diet, often only dry foods and very little fruit or vegetables. There is often an association with smell and touch hypersensitivity, e.g. avoidance of messy play, and improvement is slow over time. Encouraging playing with food, other messy play and regular times outside of meal to try new foods may be of benefit. There may not be a significant improvement in dietary variety until social pressures on eating increase in adolescence

Further reading

Emond A, Drewett R, Blair P, Emmett P. Postnatal factors associated with failure to thrive in term infants in the Avon Longitudinal Study of Parents and Children. *Arch Dis Child* 2007;92:115–119

Okoromah CA, Ekure EN, Lesi FE, Okunowo WO, Tijani BO, Okeiyi JC. Prevalence, profile and predictors of malnutrition in children with congenital heart defects: a case-control observational study. *Arch Dis Child* 2011;96:354–360

Wright CM, Parkinson KN, Drewett RF. How does maternal and child feeding behavior relate to weight gain and failure to thrive? Data from a prospective birth cohort. *Pediatrics* 2006;117:1262–1269

Food aversion

This can occur after prolonged enteral or parenteral feeding, vomiting or food anxieties in the family. It is associated with delayed weaning and autistic spectrum disorders.

Important features from history

- Prematurity, prolonged enteral feeds, intestinal failure, significant vomiting in infancy
- Patterns of family eating: eating together at a table, home cooking, snacking
- Other sensory aversion
- Parental anxiety and 'force-feeding' can exacerbate food aversion
- Family history of food aversion

Differential diagnosis

- Primary sensory aversion: isolated or part of autistic spectrum disorder
- Food aversion secondary to delayed introduction of oral feeds or persistent vomiting
- Oromotor disorder
- Cleft palate
- Foregut dysmotility with vomiting

Investigations

- Assessment by speech and language therapist (SALT), which may include videofluoroscopy for oromotor dysfunction

Practical Approach to Paediatric Gastroenterology, Hepatology and Nutrition, First Edition.
Deirdre Kelly, Ronald Bremner, Jane Hartley, and Diana Flynn.
© 2014 John Wiley & Sons, Ltd. Published 2014 by John Wiley & Sons, Ltd.

Management

- There is no specific pattern of dietary re-introduction for food aversion
- When weaning from enteral nutrition to oral diet, gradual reduction of total calories and number of hours of overnight feeding helps develop hunger and encourages eating. This should be done with the support of a multidisciplinary feeding team, including a SALT and psychology
- For more generalised sensory aversion or food neophobia, encourage gradual introduction of new foods into the diet. Use of regular food 'play' times outside regular meals can allow the child to explore new foods in a low pressure environment. Messy play is helpful for generalised sensory aversion
- Families should be encouraged to eat together and to avoid putting too much pressure on the child to eat

Further reading

Evans S, Daly A, MacDonald A, Davies P, Booth IW. Impact of nutrient density of nocturnal enteral feeds on appetite: a prospective, randomised crossover study. *Arch Dis Child* 2007;92:602–607

Shim JE, Kim J, Mathai RA; STRONG Kids Research Team. Associations of infant feeding practices and picky eating behaviors of preschool children. *J Am Diet Assoc* 2011;111:1363–1368

Wright CM, Smith KH, Morrison J. Withdrawing feeds from children on long term enteral feeding: factors associated with success and failure. *Arch Dis Child* 2011;96:433–439

Ingestion of non-food items (pica)

CHAPTER 40

Pica is the ingestion of non-food items, e.g. wallpaper, grass, hair (Table 40.1). It is more common in pre-school children. It may be associated with iron or zinc deficiency.

Presentation is variable and may be non-specific (Table 40.1). If an ingested metallic object cannot be confirmed as lead free, lead levels must be checked.

Important features from history

- Autism
- Old housing (lead paint)

Red flags: Signs of trichobezoar
Gastric bezoars can lead to: • Gastric ulcers and perforation • Intussusception • Cholestasis • Small bowel obstruction. 90% of cases are girls <20 years of age.

Outcome

- Good outcomes can usually be achieved for bezoar removal
- Psychiatric support may be required, especially for trichotillomania.
- For lead poisoning, early recognition leads to improved outcome

Practical Approach to Paediatric Gastroenterology, Hepatology and Nutrition, First Edition.
Deirdre Kelly, Ronald Bremner, Jane Hartley, and Diana Flynn.
© 2014 John Wiley & Sons, Ltd. Published 2014 by John Wiley & Sons, Ltd.

Table 40.1 Diagnosing non-food ingestion

Diagnosis	History	Investigation	Management
Lead poisoning	Abdominal pain, vomiting, constipation, irritability, agitation, acute encephalopathy Old housing (lead paint)	FBC and film AXR stippling with lead particles Knee X-ray: lead lines Blood lead level (investigate further if >1μg/mL); symptoms usually only occur if level >2.5μg/mL	Chelation therapy with dimercaprol, edetate calcium disodium or succimer if level >4.5μg/mL Endoscopic removal of upper gastrointestinal tract objects; for those beyond stomach, whole bowel irrigation with PEG Education and elimination of sources of lead
Trichobezoar (Figure 40.1)	Trichotillomania, tricophagia, vomiting, abdominal pain, ± abdominal mass	Abdominal X-ray Endoscopy Usually gastric but described in all parts of the gastrointestinal tract	Gastric: endoscopic removal with fragmentation of the bezoar Enzymatic therapy and gastric lavage may be needed Psychiatric referral to prevent recurrence
Lactobezoar	Abdominal pain and vomiting	Abdominal ultrasound Abdominal X-ray and double-contrast radiography of upper gastrointestinal tract using a non-ionic water-soluble medium with air insufflation also described	Nasogastric N-acetyl cysteine 10mg/kg in 50mL of normal saline Aspirate 6 hourly, until no milk curds visible and dissolution confirmed on ultrasound

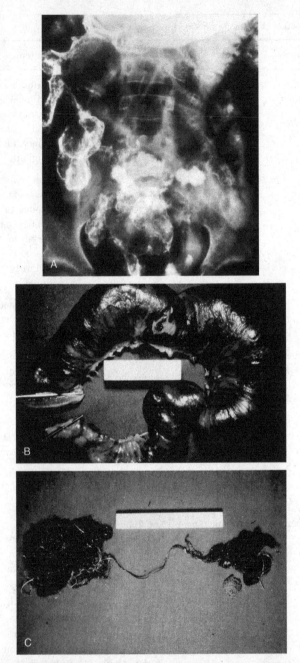

Figure 40.1 (A) Barium study of patient with recurrent vomiting and abdominal pain and three episodes of intussusception showing multiple filling defects and an unusual radiological picture. (B) Laparotomy revealed gangrenous ileo-ileal intussusceptions. (C) The lumen was occluded by swallowed hair, string and wool.

Further reading

Gonuguntla V, Joshi DD. Rapunzel syndrome. *Clin Med Res* 2009;7: 99–102

Lynch KA, Feola PG, Guenther E. Gastric trichobezoar: an important cause of abdominal pain presenting to the pediatric emergency department. *Pediatr Emerg Care* 2003;19:343–347

VanArsdale JL, Leiker RD, Kohn M, Merritt TA, Horowitz BZ. Lead poisoning from a toy necklace. *J Pediatr* 2004;114:1096–1099

Nutrition in neurodisability

The child with a neurodisability is at high risk of gastrointestinal complications, in particular feeding and swallowing difficulties (Table 41.1). Children with cerebral palsy have a high rate of feeding difficulties (>50%) and in those with quadriplegia this can rise to 85%.

Important features from history

- Length of meal times
- Recurrent chest infections: may indicate aspiration pneumonias
- Choking episodes

Examination

- Assessing malnutrition can be difficult, but growth charts are available for cerebral palsy and certain other neurodisabilites. Triceps skinfold thickness <10th centile is suggestive of malnutrition in cerebral palsy
- Examination for nutrition should include limb perfusion and muscle strength, including ability to cough and use accessory muscles of respiration

Management

- If meals usually take >30 minutes, then consider gastrostomy with oral feeds limited to 20–30 minutes
- In the presence of an unsafe swallow, then a gastrostomy ± fundoplication should be performed, following a trial of nasogastric feeding (see Chapter 49)

Practical Approach to Paediatric Gastroenterology, Hepatology and Nutrition, First Edition. Deirdre Kelly, Ronald Bremner, Jane Hartley, and Diana Flynn. © 2014 John Wiley & Sons, Ltd. Published 2014 by John Wiley & Sons, Ltd.

Table 41.1 Factors that may affect feeding in children with neurodisability

Feature	Presentation	Investigation	Management
Unsafe swallow	Drooling, choking on feeds, aspiration	SALT assessment with videofluoroscopy Chest X-ray	Use enteral feeding
Delayed swallow	Pooling of secretions in mouth	SALT assessment with videofluoroscopy	May require thickened liquids Slow oral feeding
Foregut dysmotility	Regurgitation, vomiting, aspiration	pH study Chest X-ray Upper gastrointestinal tract contrast study to exclude malrotation	Antireflux agents Consider jejunal feeding/ fundoplication
Constipation	Vomiting; poor appetite	Per rectal examination Abdominal X-ray (if uncertainty)	Laxatives High fibre feed

SALT, salt and language therapist.

- Gastro-oesophageal reflux should be treated medically before consideration of fundoplication, unless there is significant aspiration due to reflux (see Chapter 3)
- Vomiting in cerebral palsy may be secondary to abnormal vomiting reflex with forceful vomiting, excess salivation or retching. If there is considerable retching, then a fundoplication may not prevent this from continuing

Outcome

With good nutrition medical complications are reduced, with fewer hospital admissions and improved family quality of life.

Further reading

Srinivasan R, Irvine T, Dalzell M. Indications for percutaneous endoscopic gastrostomy and procedure-related outcome. *J Pediatr Gastroenterol Nutr* 2009;49:584–588

Sullivan PB (ed). Feeding and Nutrition in Children with Neurodevelopmental Disabilities. London: Mac Keith Press, 2009

Turck D, Michaud L. Growth in children with neurological impairments. *J Pediatr Gastroenterol Nutr* 2010;51:S143–S144

Malnutrition

Malnutrition in children due to lack of food is rare in the UK. Most undernutrition is related to chronic illness, with around 10–20% of hospitalised children at risk (Table 42.1). Serial height and weight plots may aid earlier identification in vulnerable children.

Eating disorders in young children are uncommon (incidence 3 per 100 000).

Important features from history

- Sudden weight loss
- Drooling, coughing, choking, dysphagia and/or food impaction
- Vomiting, abdominal pain, diarrhoea
- Heartburn and dyspepsia
- Fever
- Thirst and increased urination
- Known food allergy
- Concerns about body image
- Factitious illness may present with poor feeding
- Liver disease

Examination

- Jaundice, hepatosplenomegaly: liver disease
- Fullness and tenderness in right iliac fossa: –terminal ileal Crohn's, lymphoma
- Epigastric tenderness: gastritis
- Cold peripheries, lanugo, bradycardia, postural hypotension: eating disorder

Practical Approach to Paediatric Gastroenterology, Hepatology and Nutrition, First Edition.
Deirdre Kelly, Ronald Bremner, Jane Hartley, and Diana Flynn.
© 2014 John Wiley & Sons, Ltd. Published 2014 by John Wiley & Sons, Ltd.

Table 42.1 Common diagnoses associated with malnutrition

Diagnosis	Presentation
Inflammatory bowel disease	Abdominal pain
	Diarrhoea (± blood)
	Faltering linear growth
	Delayed puberty
Helicobacter pylori	Vomiting
	Nausea
	Dyspepsia
	Epigastric tenderness
Coeliac disease	Presentation varies with age (see Chapter 12) and may include abdominal pain, vomiting, diarrhoea
Eosinophilic oesophagitis	Dysphagia
	Abdominal pain
	Food impaction
	Known allergy/atopy
Eating disorder (see Information: Eating disorders)	Loss of appetite
	Altered body image
	Cold peripheries
	Lanugo
	Bradycardia
Autistic spectrum disorder	Food restriction and 'faddy' eating
	Sensory aversion
Diabetes mellitus	Excessive thirst
	Increased urination
	Abdominal pain
Chronic liver disease (see Chapter 24)	Poor weight gain
	Pruritis
	Fat-soluble vitamin deficiency
	Bleeding from gums and bruising

- Poor dentition: coeliac, bulimia nervosa
- Marks on knuckles: evidence of self-induced vomiting
- Hepatosplenomegaly, lymphadenopathy: malignancy, e.g. lymphoma, leukaemia

Investigations

- Baseline nutrition screen: including U&E, calcium, phosphate, magnesium, CRP, trace elements (copper, selenium, zinc), fat-soluble vitamins (A, D, E, PT), ferritin, glucose
- Urine for glucose, ketones
- See Gastroenterology and Hepatology sections for named gastrointestinal/liver diseases
- For immune deficiency disorders see Chapter 9

Management

- Management plans for chronic diseases should specifically consider nutrition with the support of a dietitian or/nutritional support team
- Depending on the cause, treatment may include advice on calorie-dense foods and use of extra fat mixed with foods to increase calorie intake without the need to substantially increase volume of food intake. If this is insufficient, then nutritional supplements may be used, although these may further reduce food intake by further appetite suppression. Enteral feeds, usually overnight, or even parenteral nutritional support may be required
- Note that in severe and acute malnutrition refeeding syndrome is a possibility Vitamin and mineral deficiencies may accompany malnutrition (Table 42.2)

Table 42.2 Features of vitamin deficiency in malnutrition

	Deficiency seen especially in	Specific deficiency	Symptoms/signs
Vitamin			
Fat-soluble vitamins (A, D, E, K)	Fat malabsorption including cystic fibrosis, cholestasis, short bowel syndrome	Vitamin A	Night blindness Hyperkeratosis Xerophthalmia, Impaired immunity

(Continued)

Table 42.2 (*Continued*)

	Deficiency seen especially in	Specific deficiency	Symptoms/signs
		Vitamin D	Rickets
			Ostemalacia
			Congenital rickets if mother deficient
		Vitamin E	Haemolytic anaemia of the newborns
			Peripheral neuropathy
			Muscle weakness
			Ophthalmoplegia
		Vitamin K	Haemorrhagic disease of the newborn
			Other bleeding, e.g. gums
			Bony weakness
Vitamin B_{12}	Terminal ileal disease/ resection		Anaemia
			Depression
	Gastric atrophy with decreased intrinsic factor		Subacute combined degeneration of the cord
	Pernicious anaemia		
Vitamin C	Malnutrition		Scurvy
	Malabsorption		Poor wound healing
			Bruising
			Skin changes
			Eventually heart failure, oedema and seizures

Table 42.2 (Continued)

	Deficiency seen especially in	Specific deficiency	Symptoms/signs
Mineral			
Zinc	Short bowel syndrome	Acrodermatitis enteropathica	Severe skin rash in nappy area, face
	After gastric disconnect surgery	Note also occurs as a known rare recessive disorder	Diarrhoea
			Poor wound healing
	Gut inflammation		Photophobia
			Increased infection risk
Copper		Bariatric surgery	Pancytopaenia
		X-linked Menke's disease	Osteoporosis
			Separation of the epiphysis
Selenium		Keshan disease in areas of selenium-poor soil	Cardiomyopathy
			Skeletal myopathy

Information: Eating disorders

NB: It is important to first exclude any underlying disease process

Investigations
- Lying and standing blood pressure for postural hypotension
- ECG, U&E, phosphate and magnesium
- Baseline inflammatory markers, thyroid function and calprotectin

Management
- Refer to a child and adolescent psychiatrist within an eating disorders team
- Admission to a specialised unit may be necessary for structured food re-introduction and family support

(Continued)

- Admission to medical ward: consider if high medical risk (see Red flags for Junior MARSIPAN). Medical admissions require strict dietary supervision, regular fluid and electrolyte monitoring for refeeding syndrome, cardiac monitoring and a mental health nurse to support high risk children, e.g. suicidal ideation

Note: children with eating disorders may demonstrate manipulative behaviours. A consistent plan known by all members of staff and parents is important, including exact portion size, mealtime monitoring (including 30 minutes after the meal – risk of self-induced emesis).

Red flags: Eating disorders

Junior MARSIPAN for red amber and green categorisation http://www .rcpsych.ac.uk/files/pdfversion/CR168.pdf)

Note that the highest risk for sudden death is a BMI or weight for height % <70%.

This latter can be calculated from:

current BMI × 100)/BMI of 50th centile for child's age

Information: Nutrition in children on chemotherapy

Oral mucositis: the oral mucosa has a very high mitotic index and therefore is at high risk of mucositis with chemotherapy, with oral ulceration and inflammation. The pain can be severe enough to require opioids and often prevents children from eating.

Refeeding syndrome

Refeeding syndrome occurs in children treated for acute severe malnutrition or chronic malnutrition (Algorithm 42.1). It can occur with oral, enteral or parenteral feeding.

Red flags: Signs of refeeding

- Early signs are non-specific
- Regular measurements of serum electrolytes for fall in phosphate and magnesium and ECG monitoring if phosphate levels <0.5 mmol/L
- Other early signs include confusion, muscle weakness and heart failure

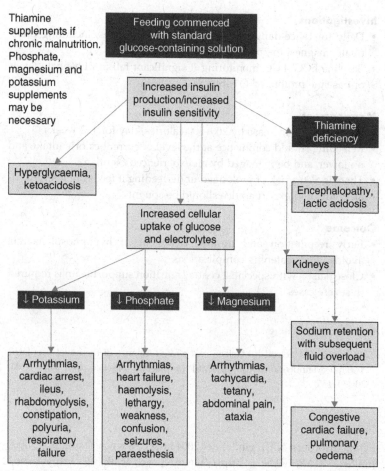

Algorithm 42.1 Complications of refeeding

Information: Effect of starvation on metabolism

- Once glycogen stores are exhausted there is no readily available glucose supply so energy is produced from skeletal muscle breakdown
- Subsequent fatty acid lipolysis produces ketone bodies
- Insulin production falls due to low carbohydrate intake
- Circulating concentrations of electrolytes, particularly phosphate, are maintained at the expense of intracellular stores

Investigations

- Daily (or twice-daily) measurement of electrolytes, including phosphate, magnesium, potassium and sodium
- Baseline ECG: ECG monitoring if significant fall in phosphate levels or baseline prolonged QT interval

Management

- Staged calorie increase by 200–300 calories/day for 1–2 weeks
- Refeeding should commence at the level of current calorie intake and no lower, and be managed by an experienced dietitian
- There is also a risk of prolonged underfeeding if feeds are inappropriately low and expert advice should be sought

Outcome

- Early recognition and prompt treatment of hypophosphataemia avoids life-threatening complications
- Close liaison with specialist centre/nutrition support team is required in severe cases

Further reading

Gerasimidis K, Macleod I, Maclean A *et al*. Performance of the novel Paediatric Yorkhill Malnutrition Score (PYMS) in hospital practice. *Clin Nutr* 2011; 30:430–435

Key web links

Eating disorders: NICE guidelines 2004 http://www.nice.org.uk/CG009
Junior MARSIPAN: http://www.rcpsych.ac.uk/files/pdfversion/CR168.pdf

Obesity

Childhood obesity is part of a global epidemic. Over 25% of children in the UK are overweight, and this is expected to rise to over 50% by 2020. Weight gain occurs as a result of a positive energy balance, i.e. eating more calories than are expended. Medications, genetic disorders and physical immobility increase the risk of obtaining a positive balance.

Body mass index (BMI) [weight (kg)/height (m^2)] varies with age and gender. The child's BMI must be plotted on a BMI chart. In clinical practice, generally a BMI >91st centile and >98th centile is recognised as being overweight and obese, respectively. Severe obesity is defined as a BMI >99.6th centile, with very severe and extreme obesity defined a BMI >3.5 SD (standard deviation) and >4 SD, respectively (RCPCH UK 2013 charts).

Obesity is classified as primary (pathological) or secondary (simple) (Table 43.1). Secondary obesity may be amenable to treatment.

Important features from history

- Age of onset of obesity: early onset associated with genetic causes
- Congenital anomalies, e.g. polydactyly, Bardot–Biedl
- Hypotonia: Prader–Willi syndrome
- Learning difficulties
- Dietary history: be thorough
- Physical activity: frequency, duration, intensity
- Growth: underlying cause for obesity, e.g. endocrine dysfunction
- Polyuria/polydipsia: type 2 diabetes
- Family history: obesity, type 2 diabetes, hypertension
- Sleeping problems: snoring, restlessness after sleep, lethargy

Practical Approach to Paediatric Gastroenterology, Hepatology and Nutrition, First Edition.
Deirdre Kelly, Ronald Bremner, Jane Hartley, and Diana Flynn.
© 2014 John Wiley & Sons, Ltd. Published 2014 by John Wiley & Sons, Ltd.

Table 43.1 Comparison of simple and pathological obesity

Simple obesity	Pathological obesity
Common	Rare
Strong family history	Family history: rare
Tall stature	Short stature
Normal physical examination	Dysmorphic features and other stigmata
Normal development	Developmental delay

Examination

- Height and weight, BMI
- Dysmorphic features – syndromes:
  - Chromosomal, e.g. 1p36 deletion
  - Prader–Willi syndrome
  - Down's syndrome
- Distribution of adiposity:
  - Central/cushingoid
  - Striae: can occur in obesity and not only with Cushing's syndrome
- Acanthosis nigricans: darkened and thickened skin around neck and axillae; marker of insulin resistance
- Blood pressure: use appropriate sized cuff
- Visual fields/cranial nerves: may indicate pituitary abnormality

Investigations (Algorithm 43.1)

- Urea and electrolytes
- Calcium and phosphate (parathyroid hormone, PTH)
- Thyroid function tests
- Fasting lipids
- Liver function tests: transaminases
- Oral glucose tolerance test
- Sleep study
- Dexamethasone test: if concerned re Cushing's
- Genetics of obesity study (GOOS, Cambridge)
- Liver ultrasound: elevated transaminases
- Ambulatory blood pressure

Management

Management of obesity is still suboptimal. Strategies for weight reduction include dietary advice and support, and programmes to increase

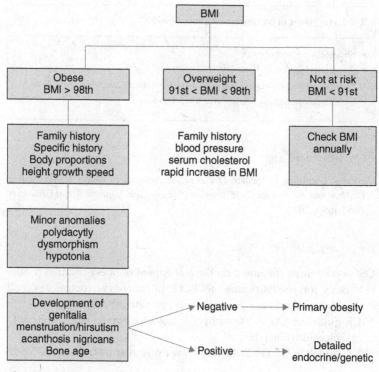

Algorithm 43.1 Investigation of obesity

exercise and decrease time in front of computer and TV screens. In morbid obesity, bariatric surgery and laparoscopic sleeve gastrectomy have been used in adolescence. However, complications include trace element deficiency and increased suicide risk has been described in adults.

- Patient education
- Mainstay of treatment is lifestyle changes:
  - Change in eating patterns: healthy eating
  - Appropriate portion size
  - Reduce sedentary behaviour and increase physical activity
- Drugs – limited:
  - Orilistat (lipase inhibitor) may help to reduce weight
- Poorly tolerated side-effects: flatulence, diarrhoea, steatorrhoea
- Bariatric surgery: considered in post-pubertal adolescents with extreme obesity when lifestyle changes have failed. Must be carried out only after extensive evaluation in a specialised centre

> **Red flags: When to be concerned about obesity**
>
> - Short stature and obesity
> - Associated learning disability
> - Positive screen for co-morbidities: acanthosis nigricans, sleep problems, hypertension, non-alcoholic fatty liver disease

Further reading

Gibson P, Edmunds L, Haslam DW *et al. An Approach to Weight Management in Children and Adolescents (2–18 Years) in Primary Care.* London: Royal College of Paediatrics, 2002

Key web links

OSCA consensus statement on the assessment of obese children & adolescents for paediatricians –RCPCH: http://www.rcpch.ac.uk/child-health/standards-care/nutrition-and-growth/obesity/obesity

NICE guideline CG43 2006: http://www.nice.org.uk/nicemedia/pdf/cg43niceguideline.pdf

SIGN guideline 115 Feb 2010: http://www.sign.ac.uk/pdf/sign115.pdf

Intestinal failure

Intestinal failure (IF) occurs where absorption of nutrients and water from the gut is inadequate to provide sufficient nutrition for maintenance and growth, resulting in the need for parenteral nutrition (PN). Causes include short bowel syndrome, enterocyte abnormalities and dysmotility syndromes.

Information: Classification of intestinal failure

- Type I: self-limiting, resolution expected within 4 weeks
- Type II: medium term, resolves within weeks to months but before the need for home parenteral nutrition (HPN)
- Type III: irreversible/long term, usually requires HPN

Important features in the history

- Family history
- Duration of symptoms
- Degree of weight loss
- Evidence of dehydration
- Recurrent infections/evidence of immune system defects

Baseline investigations

- Nutritional bloods, including:
  - U&E, calcium, magnesium and phosphate
  - LFTs

Practical Approach to Paediatric Gastroenterology, Hepatology and Nutrition, First Edition.
Deirdre Kelly, Ronald Bremner, Jane Hartley, and Diana Flynn.
© 2014 John Wiley & Sons, Ltd. Published 2014 by John Wiley & Sons, Ltd.

- ○ FBC and coagulation: fat soluble vitamin
- ○ B vitamins, folate and ferritin, triglycerides
- Strict fluid balance: record stools, vomiting and other losses, e.g. chest drain
- May need brief urinary catheterisation to assess urine output accurately if very watery diarrhoea
- Anthropometry, including head circumference <1-year old
- Urinary electrolytes: to determine adequate sodium input

General management and adaptation

PN should be started when there the gut is unable to provide nutrition for a period of at least a week, or even shorter where there is already significant malnutrition. It should not be used where sufficient nutrition can be given enterally or where the period of non-feeding is likely to be only a few days.

Consider refeeding syndrome if significant weight loss (see Chapter 42).

Trophic feeding

Enterocytes require enteral nutrition for optimal growth and health, so even small amounts of feed given continuously will be beneficial. In young infants this can be as little as 1 mL/hour and around 5 mL/hour in an older child.

- Slow introduction of continuous enteral feeding, progressing to introduction of small oral boluses
- Proton pump inhibitors decrease volume of gastric secretions
- Consider jejunal feeding if foregut dysmotility
- Antimotility agents such as loperamide for diarrhoea (if colon present)
- Cycled enteral antibiotics for bacterial overgrowth

When to refer to nutrition support team (NST)

All children with type II intestinal failure require multidisciplinary input from the NST for ongoing support and planning for home PN if necessary. Once it is recognised that a child is likely to have a long-term PN requirement for permanent intestinal failure or severe short bowel syndrome, referral should not be delayed.

The NST also provides support in the nutritional management of any child with complex nutritional needs, especially where there are complicating factors such as fluid balance and difficulty establishing enteral or oral feeding.

Table 44.1 Normal bowel lengths at different ages	
Age	Bowel length (ligament of Treitz to ileo-caecal valve)
Premature infant	Correlates to gestational age and doubles in length from 28 weeks to term
Term infant	240 cm
15 years old	430 cm
Adult	600–2000cm

Short bowel syndrome (SBS)

Normal bowel length varies with age and increases maximally over the first year of life (Table 44.1). SBS in children is most common in infancy and is defined as a bowel length of <80 cm, with very short bowel defined as <40 cm and extreme as <15 cm.

Important features from history
- Length of remaining bowel: <40 cm is likely to require HPN
- Calibre and motility of remaining bowel
- Part of bowel remaining: ileum more likely to adapt than jejunum; colon is important for water reabsorption and nutrient production from short chain fatty acids
- If the ileo-caecal valve has been removed, there is increased risk of bacterial overgrowth

Management and adaptation (Algorithm 44.1 and Table 44.2)
Adaptation is the process by which intestinal hypertrophy and hyperplasia allows increased nutrient and water absorption.

Threshold is the volume of feed after which bowel can longer absorb nutrients and/or water resulting in development of diarrhoea ± vomiting.

Information: Non-transplant surgery for short bowel syndrome

- Aim is to decrease the calibre of dilated bowel loops, to improve stasis and decrease bacterial overgrowth, and to increase length and absorptive capacity
- Tapering procedure: if bacterial overgrowth but increased bowel length not required

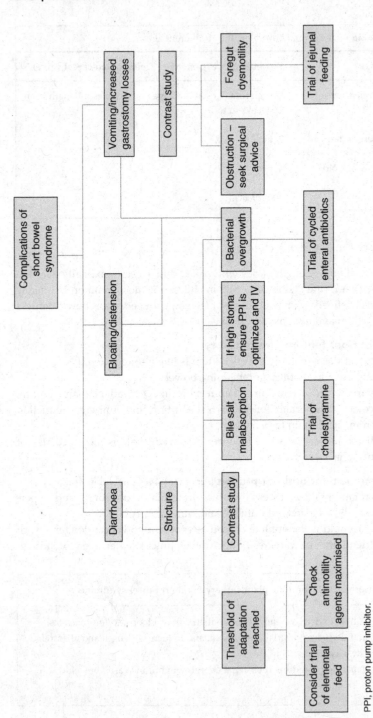

PPI, proton pump inhibitor.

Algorithm 44.1 Management strategies in short bowel syndrome

Table 44.2 Conditions giving rise to short bowel syndrome and management

Diagnosis	Aetiology	Particular complications
Necrotising enterocolitis (NEC)	Premature babies (especially <1500 g) Gram-negative sepsis Hypoxia Altered intestinal blood flow	Total gut ischaemia
Cardiac NEC	Seen after bypass for cardiac surgery	Protein-losing enteropathy, e.g. after Fontan
Gastroschisis	? Association with recreational drug use	Often poorer outcome, especially if other anomalies present Dilated and dysmotile bowel
Neonatal volvulus/atresias	Some genetic cases of malrotation, including *FOXF1* transcription factor mutations There are also four syndromes featuring malrotation	Motility often disordered Perforation of bowel *in utero* with meconium peritonitis and/or hydrops fetalis
Congenital short bowel	Unknown; very rare Some cases familial May be associated with other anomalies	Usually associated with malrotation
Meconium ileus (MI)/Distal Intestinal Obstruction Syndrome (DIOS)	Often associated with cystic fibrosis Simple or complex, i.e. associated with atresia, perforation, etc.	About half of patients with and most with DIOS respond to conservative treatment Complications include volvulus, atresia or perforation

(Continued)

Table 44.2 (*Continued*)

Diagnosis	Aetiology	Particular complications
Crohn's disease	After multiple resections	Ongoing disease activity
Ischaemia	Drugs, e.g. cocaine	
	Malignancy	
	Mesenteric vascular ischaemia	
	Vasculitis	
Malignancy	E.g. lymphoma	Enteric infection, e.g. adenovirus, *Clostridium difficile*

Outcome

This has improved significantly in recent years, with the use of early IV antibiotics for central line infections, prophylaxis with antibacterial line locks and improved PN provision to decrease liver disease. The need for small bowel transplantation can be avoided in most children.

Enteropathy

Most congenital enteropathies present in the first 6 months of life, often in the first weeks (Table 44.3). Others may be unmasked later or develop gradually over the first year or two of life.

Red flags: Pitfalls in diagnosis of diarrhoea
Severe watery diarrhoea may be mistaken for urine and children may present with dehydration

Important features from history
- Genetic factors: consanguinity, previous neonatal deaths
- Antenatal history: polyhydramnios
- Recurrent infections: immune deficiency

Table 44.3 Types of enteropathies presenting in infancy

Type	Specific disease	Investigation
Immune	Autoimmune enteropathy, e.g. IPEX, SCID, CVID, AIDS	CD4/CD8 counts
		Functional antibodies
		Complement
		Lymphocyte subsets
		Autoantibodies (parietal cell, goblet cell)
		FOXP3 mutation
Enterocyte abnormalities	MVID	Endoscopy and biopsies, including electron microscopy
	Tufting enteropathy	
Congenital salt-losing diarrhoeas	Chloride-losing diarrhoea	Stool electrolytes
	Sodium-losing diarrhoea	
Disaccharidase deficiency	Sucrose–isomaltase deficiency	Endoscopy and biopsies for disaccharidases
	Glucose-galactose deficiency	
Allergic	Cow's milk protein intolerance	Trial of dairy free diet
		Endoscopy and biopsies
	Eosinophilic enteropathy	
Fat malabsorption	Cystic fibrosis	IRT/sweat test
	Pancreatic insufficiency: Schwachmann	Barium meal and follow-through
	Intestinal lymphangiectasia	Stool elastase

AIDS, acquired immune deficiency syndrome; CVID, common variable immunodeficiency; IPEX, immunodysregulation polyendocrinopathy enteropathy X-linked syndrome; IRT, immunoreactive trypsinogen; MVID, microvillous inclusion disease; SCID, severe combined immunodeficiency.

Table 44.4 Investigation of enteropathy

Investigation	Outcome
Stool electrolytes and osmolality	Secretory versus osmotic diarrhoea (see Chapter 9). Secretory diarrhoea does not stop on stopping enteral intake and fluid requirements are likely to be high
Stool alpha-1-antitrypsin	Protein-losing enteropathy
Stool chymotrypsin/elastase	Fat malabsorption

Investigations

These are listed in Table 44.4.

Management

Diarrhoea is usually the main limitation to advancing enteral feeds. Antimotility agents may be tried:

- Loperamide starting at 0.5 mg/kg/day or less in four divided doses can be increased slowly to 1 mg/kg/day
- Codeine phosphate can also be used, but may cause vomiting

For autoimmune enteropathies, immunosuppression or occasionally bone marrow transplantation may be employed.

Outcome

The outcome for children with enteropathy depends on the underlying cause, and some children may require life-long PN, with others able to wean completely onto enteral feeds. Repeated trials of enteral tolerance with gradual increase in enteral feeds can often result in significant decreases in PN requirements over time. Small bowel transplantation or bone marrow transplantation may need to be considered.

Pseudo-obstruction

Chronic intestinal pseudo-obstruction syndrome (CIPOS) results from impaired intestinal motility with signs of obstruction in the absence of mechanical occlusion.

Primary CIPOS may be familial or sporadic, due to abnormalities in enteric smooth muscle (visceral myopathy) or the enteric nervous system (visceral neuropathy) (Table 44.5). In myopathies other smooth muscle-containing organs may be affected.

Secondary CIPOS may occur at any age.

Table 44.5 Types of pseudo-obstruction

Disorder	Features
Neurogenic	
Hirschsprung's disease (aganglionosis) (<1% whole bowel affected; 80% only part of colon affected)	Failure of migration of ganglion cells to affect variable length of gastrointestinal tract
	Absence of myenteric and submucosal plexus
	Incidence 1 in 5000
	M > F
	Delayed passage of meconium
	Risk of enterocolitis
	Hearing loss, abnormal pigmentation in some patients
	In 20% of Hirschsprung's cases, there are associated abnormalities: • Trisomy 21 • Waardenburg–Shah syndrome • Neurocristopathy syndromes • Piebaldism • Multiple endocrine neoplasia type II
Intestinal neuronal dysplasias (hypoganglionosis or hyperganglionosis)	Delayed maturation of enteric nervous system
	Clinically similar to Hirschsprung's but may have milder features
Familial visceral neuropathy	Heterogeneous
	Abnormalities of myenteric plexus
	Associated with achalasia
Myopathic	
Familial visceral myopathy (FVM)	Autosomal recessive or dominant
	Atrophy and fibrosis of the muscularis propria
	May involve other organs, e.g. eye, urinary tract and peripheral nerves

(Continued)

Table 44.5 (*Continued*)

Disorder	Features
Mitochondrial disease involving skeletal muscle (ragged red fibres) Mitochondrial neurogastrointestinal encephalopathy (MNGIE) syndrome	Multisystem mitochondrial disease Gastrointestinal dysmotility with pseudo-obstruction Peripheral neuropathy and myopathy Ophthalmoplegia
X-linked intestinal pseudo-obstruction	Mutations in *FLNA*, the gene encoding filamin A, a cytoskeletal protein
Hormonal and other causes	
Neural crest tumours	Rarely can give rise to symptoms of pseudo-obstruction
Leiomyositis	Very rare. May be history of autoimmune disease
Drugs: vincristine	Rare but consider in children with abdominal pain and constipation following chemotherapy
Prune belly syndrome	1 in 35000–50000 95% males Absent abdominal muscles Bilateral cryptorchidism, renal tract abnormalities and UTIs Risk of antenatal volvulus, atresias Pulmonary, skeletal and cardiac defects possible
Megacystis–microcolon–intestinal hypoperistalsis syndrome (MMIH)	? Autosomal recessive but female to male ratio 4:1 Megacystis, hydronephrosis and UTIs Microcolon and distal microileum, gut malrotation Intestinal hypoperistalsis

UTI, urinary tract infection.

Important features from history
- Constipation: often severe, i.e. no bowel movement for >2–3 weeks
- Vomiting
- Abdominal pain and distension
- Episodes of diarrhoea (enteritis)
- Food intolerance and weight loss
- Antenatal: bladder abnormalities on scan

Investigations
- Abdominal X-ray
- Contrast follow through or enema: exclude atresia/stricture
- Rectal suction biopsy and full thickness intestinal : determine extent of disease
- Autoantibodies, including ANCA, DNA, ANA, SMA
- Manometry: may help distinguish between neuropathic and myopathic forms and demonstrates tone, phasic pressure and compliance of the colon; in the small bowel amplitude of contractions are demonstrated
- Nuclear medicine: gastric emptying studies – foregut dysmotility

Management
- Parenteral nutrition
- Cycled enteral antibiotics for bacterial overgrowth in dilated bowel loops
- Motility agents, e.g. domperidone
- Gastric and/or ileal decompression: gastrostomy with venting; ileostomy may decrease bowel dilatation, thus improving function
- Immunosuppression may be indicated in autoimmune myocyte destruction

---

Information: Acute colonic pseudo-obstruction (ACPO)

Can occur with trauma, electrolyte disturbances, medications affecting gastrointestinal motility (such as vincristine and opioids) and sepsis. Ischaemia and perforation may ensue.

Management
- Bowel rest and avoidance of laxatives (especially lactulose which may increase bacterial proliferation)
- Treatment with neostigmine has been reported

Complications

As for PN, plus:
- High rate of stoma prolapse in CIPOS
- Enterocolitis in Hirschsprung's

Outcome

As for all long-term PN patients, outcome has improved over time with better line care and sepsis prevention and management. Newer therapies such as stem cell transplantation are still some way off.

Red flags: Kawasaki disease

- Kawasaki disease presenting as acute obstruction
- Consider Kawasaki disease where there is acute pseudo-obstruction and fever

---

Further reading

Duro D, Kamin D, Duggan C. Overview of pediatric short bowel syndrome. *J Pediatr Gastroenterol Nutr* 2008;47:S33–S36

Di Lorenzo C, Youssef NN. Diagnosis and management of intestinal motility disorders. *Semin Pediatr Surg* 2010;19:50–58

Khalil BA, Ba'ath ME, Aziz A *et al.* Intestinal rehabilitation and bowel reconstructive surgery: improved outcomes in children with short bowel syndrome. *J Pediatr Gastroenterol Nutr* 2012;54:505–509

Ruemmele FM, Moes N, de Serre NP, Rieux-Laucat F, Goulet O. Clinical and molecular aspects of autoimmune enteropathy and immune dysregulation, polyendocrinopathy autoimmune enteropathy X-linked syndrome. *Curr Opin Gastroenterol* 2008;24(6):742–748

Key web links

Intestinal failure: recommendations for tertiary management of infants and children. A Report by the Intestinal Failure Working Group, BSPGHAN and BAPS;
http://www.bspghan.org.uk/Word%20docs%20and%20PDFs/ IFWGreportfinalMar2007.pdf

NICE guidance on STEP procedure: http://guidance.nice.org.uk/IPG232

STEP registry: http://www.childrenshospital.org/cfapps/step/index .cfm

Parenteral nutrition: initiating and monitoring

The aim of parenteral nutrition is the provision of balanced intravenous nutrition support to achieve normal nutritional status and growth.

Indications

- Intestinal immaturity (premature babies)
- Intestinal failure or inability to use the intestine to support nutrition for a predicted period of at least 7 days

Commencing parenteral nutrition

Baseline requirements:
- Ensure secure central venous access: with a dedicated line for PN use only. Peripherally inserted central catheter (PICC) lines or central venous lines are both suitable. Peripheral access for PN is not advised as glucose concentration must be restricted to <12.5%
- Baseline anthropometry: height, weight [and occipitofrontal cortex (OFC) <2 years]
- Baseline bloods: U&E, LFTs, calcium, phosphate and magnesium
- Urinary electrolytes

Commence PN slowly, increasing carbohydrate and lipid concentrations over the first few days with regular electrolyte and triglyceride monitoring.

Calculating requirements: See ESPGHAN and local guidelines.

Practical Approach to Paediatric Gastroenterology, Hepatology and Nutrition, First Edition.
Deirdre Kelly, Ronald Bremner, Jane Hartley, and Diana Flynn.
© 2014 John Wiley & Sons, Ltd. Published 2014 by John Wiley & Sons, Ltd.

Information: Triglycerides and parenteral nutrition

- Triglycerides (TG) and parenteral nutrition: reduce dose of lipids if concentrations >25 mg/mL in infant or >40 mg/mL in older children
- If hypertriglyceridaemia: increase lipids by 0.5 g/kg/day and monitor TGs
- Note high risk for raised TGs: ELBW infants, sepsis and critical illness, higher lipid dose

Hypertriglyceridaemia
- Acute rises in triglycerides increases left ventricular contractility and can induce acute pancreatitis
- Risk for sepsis, diabetes and liver damage, and can be associated with hyperglycaemia, as excess carbohydrate can be converted to fatty acids
- If acute and severe, insulin has been used to treat

Parenteral nutrition components

NB: see ESPGHAN guidelines for detailed overview of PN components and use, and cautions including manganese and aluminium toxicity.
- PN consists of a complex mixture of macro- and micro-nutrients.
- Most hospitalised children's needs will be met by about 100–120% of resting energy expenditure, which may need to rise to 130–150% if malnourished (see ESPGHAN guidelines for PN)
- Lipids are more calorie dense than glucose and allow smaller total volumes of fluid for the same total calorie intake, and a lower total osmotic load
- Balancing lipid and carbohydrate helps prevent hepatic steatosis, as too high a glucose load results in lipogenesis and impaired protein metabolism, and high lipid dosing is associated with intestinal failure-associated liver disease (IFALD)
- Amino acids are needed to maintain positive nitrogen balance

Protein (Table 45.1)
- Provided as amino acid solution
- Mixture of essential/non-essential/conditionally essential amino acids for protein synthesis
- A minimum of 1–1.5 g/kg to prevent a negative nitrogen balance; max 4 g/kg/day in premature babies decreasing to about 2 g/kg/day in older children

Table 45.1 Amino acid preparations for parenteral nutrition

Amino acid	Note
Vaminolact	Neonatal/paediatric presentation based on amino acid profile of breast milk
Primene	Neonatal/paediatric presentation based on amino acid profile of cord blood
Vamin	Adult presentations of amino acids available in a range of concentrations: used in older children
Braun amino acid/others	
Synthamin	

Table 45.2 Lipid preparations for parenteral nutrition

Lipid	Main fat components
Intralipid	100% soyabean oil
Omegaven	100% fish oil
SMOF	30% soya, 30% MCT, 25% olive oil, 14% fish oil
Lipofundin	100% soyabean oil
Lipofundin MCT	50% soya, 50% MCT

MCT, medium-chain triglyceride.

Carbohydrate
- Provided as glucose; main energy source in PN
- Avoid glucose >18 g/kg/day in infants (may induce lipogenesis and contribute to hepatic steatosis; increase CO_2 production and minute volume and impair protein metabolism.)
- Watch for hyper- and hypo-glycaemia: a step-down may be required when stopping PN if cycled due to hypoglycaemia with subsequent rebound hyperglycaemia

Fat (Table 45.2)
Provided as lipids
- Non-carbohydrate source of energy and source of essential fatty acids
- Provides 25–50% of calories, limited to 3–4 g/kg/day in infants and 2–3 g/kg/day in older children

Table 45.3 Trace element preparations for parenteral nutrition

Trace element	Note
Peditrace	Paediatric presentation of trace elements
Additrace	Adult presentation of trace elements used in older children
Decan	

Table 45.4 Vitamin preparations for parenteral nutrition

Vitamin	Note
Solivito N	Neonatal/paediatric presentation of water-soluble vitamins
Vitlipid N Infant	Neonatal/paediatric presentation of fat-soluble vitamins
Vitlipid N Adult	Adult presentation of fat-soluble vitamins: used in older children
Cernevit	Combined water- and fat-soluble presentation used in adults and older children

- NB: to prevent IFALD in children on long-term PN, total lipid should be kept to <2.5 g/kg where possible and cycled to 3–5 days per week

Trace elements (Table 45.3)
- Essential micronutrients required in many metabolic processes
- Includes chromium, copper, iodine, manganese, molybdenum, selenium and zinc

Vitamins (Table 45.4)
- Essential for growth and development
- Fat-soluble vitamins: vitamins A, D, E, K
- Water-soluble vitamins: vitamins C, B (thiamine, riboflavin, pyridoxine, cobalamin, niacin, pantothenic acid, biotin, folic acid)

Electrolytes and minerals
- Essential/semi-essential for normal function and losses
- Included as a range of preparations containing sodium, chloride, potassium, calcium, magnesium, phosphate, iron and acetate

Further reading

American Society for Parenteral and Enteral Nutrition (A.S.P.E.N.) Board of Directors. Clinical Guidelines for the Use of Parenteral and Enteral Nutrition in Adult and Pediatric Patients, 2009. *J Parenter Enteral Nutr* 2009;33(3):255–259

Koletzko B, Goulet O, Hunt J, Krohn K, and Shamir R for the Parenteral Nutrition Guidelines Working Group. Guidelines on Paediatric Parenteral Nutrition of the European Society of Paediatric Gastroenterology, Hepatology and Nutrition (ESPGHAN) and the European Society for Clinical Nutrition and Metabolism (ESPEN), Supported by the European Society of Paediatric Research (ESPR). *J Pediatr Gastroenterol Nutr* 2005;41:S1–S87

Parenteral nutrition: complications

CHAPTER 46

Catheter-related bloodstream infections (CRBSI)

CRBSIs are common in infants on parenteral nutrition (PN), but decrease with age and once home parenteral nutrition (HPN) is established. The incidence of catheter-associated infection in children receiving HPN varies between 0.41 and 1.5 episodes of infection per patient year, up to 8 per 1000 catheter days, but is highest in toddlers.

The commonest infections in young children are *Staphylococcus*, *Enterococcus*, *Enterobacter*, *Klebsiella* and *Escherichia coli*, i.e. skin flora or presumed 'translocations' of enteric bacteria.

Red flags: Pitfalls in diagnosis and management of CRBSI

In infants with intestinal failure, the only signs of infection may be a drop in platelets and neutrophils and rise in bilirubin. In the presence of intestinal failure-associated liver disease (IFALD), empiric treatment with antibiotics should be considered.

Important features from history
- Fever >38°C on two occasions or >38.5°C on a single occasion
- Metabolic acidosis
- Glucose instability
- Rise in C-reactive protein (CRP)
- Systemic malaise
- Signs of severe infection: rigors, shock, collapse
- Previous infections with the same central venous line (CVL) *in situ*
- Exclude other infectious aetiology: urine, respiratory infection or even meningitis in young infants need to be considered

---

Practical Approach to Paediatric Gastroenterology, Hepatology and Nutrition, First Edition.
Deirdre Kelly, Ronald Bremner, Jane Hartley, and Diana Flynn.

Investigations

- Central and peripheral blood cultures (BC) (paired only useful if quantitative or semi-quantitative culture technique used)
- FBC, LFTs, CRP, urine culture

Management

Prompt treatment is important and may minimise liver damage.

- Broad-spectrum antibiotics until bacteria and sensitivities identified
- An individualised sepsis protocol should be established for each child with intestinal failure to tailor antibiotics as appropriate

  If necessary, remove the CVL when the following are suspected:

- Fungal infection
- *Staphylococcus aureus*
- Symptoms not settling with antibiotic therapy
- Recurrence of the same organism with the same subtype within 1 month

  Recurrent life-threatening infections, e.g. with collapse/PICU admission, is a potential indication for small bowel transplant.

Information: Prevention of CRBSI

Keys to decreased infection are:

- Management by a multidisciplinary nutrition support team
- Appropriate care bundles and training packs for patients and families
- Use of 2% chlorhexidine in isopropanol is now standard for cleaning hubs
- Use of antibacterial line locks is increasing, especially with taurolidine which prevents biofilm formation. Other agents include 70% ethanol
- Other considerations: use of single-lumen catheters dedicated to PN use; cycled enteral antibiotics to decrease bacterial overgrowth and translocation

---

Red flags: CRBSI

- Rapid deterioration is a medical emergency, and shock may develop very quickly, necessitating emergency line removal
- Consider fungal infection: where antibiotics have been used frequently, then antifungal agents should be added to protocols

Thrombosis and central venous line occlusion

CVLs are the commonest cause of venous thrombosis in children. The importance of prevention cannot be underestimated, especially in those who rely on lifelong PN.

Important features from history

- Increasing stiffness of line on flushing, increased infusion pressures, leaking from the line *or*
- Inability to withdraw blood
- Superior vena cava (SVC) syndrome (neck and face swelling together with dilated veins)
- Pain and swelling of the arm if CVL is sited in upper limbs
  Note that venous thrombosis may be asymptomatic and diagnosed by USS or MRV.

Differential diagnosis

- Blocked CVL from blood, drugs or PN within the line
- Clot or fibrin sheath in the vein
- CVL tip resting against the vein wall or compressed due to positioning or pressure from the clavicle

Investigations

- Chest X-ray to exclude CVL tip malposition or kink in the line
- A contrast line-o-gram to look for fibrin sheath or blocked line tip
- Doppler ultrasound may show extent of previous thromboses but MR venogram is more reliable for assessment of available vascular access

---

Information: Pulmonary embolus

- Rare in children
- One-third due to CVL *in situ*
- May be exacerbated by fat embolism and dehydration
- Presentation: rarely acute-onset chest pain, shortness of breath and hypoxia
- Symptoms may be mild and persist for weeks
- Atypical features: cough, haemoptysis, seizures, fever and abdominal pain, shock

Investigations
- Non-specific:
  - Elevated D-dimers, raised WBC
  - Chest X-ray
  - V/Q scan or CT angiogram
  - Pulmonary angiogram
- Thrombophilia testing for protein S and C, antithrombin III, antiphospholipid antibodies, factor V leiden, PT and APTT, prothrombin 20210 mutation, fasting homocysteine

Management
- Anticoagulation with heparin initially

Management
- Flushing between drugs and when off PN with saline. Blood sampling should be kept to a minimum
- When not in use the CVL should be flushed once to twice weekly
- Urokinase or alteplase for suspected occlusion; given as a line lock or slow infusion
- Warfarin or low molecular weight heparin for proven thrombosis; long-term therapy may be necessary
- Prevention of CVL infections

In children with extensive thrombosis, other central vessels may be used, e.g. transhepatic, azygous, right atrium. Placement should only be by an experienced operator and complications are high. Loss of vascular access is an indication for referral for small bowel transplant assessment and should be made before venous access is severely limited.

Small bowel bacterial overgrowth (SBBO)

Gut microbiotia are key players in healthy gut function. They produce short chain fatty acids which provide calories, neuro-modulatory substances and antibiotics. Alterations in gut microbiota may influence gut motility.

Information: Factors contributing to SBBO in short bowel syndrome

---

- Altered integrity of the mucosal barrier
- Stasis and dilated small bowel loops promote bacterial overgrowth
- Compromised immunity of the gut due to loss of intestinal lymphoid tissue, the effects of PN and IFALD
- Absence of the ileo-caecal valve may increase numbers of colonic species
- Proton pump inhibitors (PPIs) alter gut flora by changing acidity

---

Important features from history
- Bloating
- Diarrhoea
- Abdominal pain
- Increased CRBSI
- Weight loss

Investigations
- Hydrogen breath testing (measures bacterial fermentation products of D-glucose)

Management

- Cycled enteral antibiotics: varying regimens are used, usually with 2 weeks each of two separate antibiotics followed by 2 weeks with no antibiotics
- Domperidone to increase motility
- Surgery to reduce bowel dilatation: includes STEP procedure or tapering
- Modular feed to decrease carbohydrate and increase fat calories
- Probiotics may be of benefit

D-lactic acidosis

D-lactic acidosis is a rare complication of short bowel syndrome or other malabsorption syndromes. Carbohydrate malabsorption allows partially digested sugars to enter the colon and be metabolised by colonic bacterial flora. D-lactate is mainly produced by Gram-positive anaerobes, e.g. lactobacillus.

Important features from history

- Short bowel syndrome (SBS)/other malabsorption
- A high carbohydrate load is usual, as is decreased motility of the colon
- Encephalopathic features include: slurred speech, poor concentration, confusion, hallucinations, ataxia, nausea, aggressive behaviour and irritability
- Episodes can last from a few hours to several days and often occur in the morning following an overnight feed

Differential diagnosis

- Abnormal seizure activity
- Dumping syndrome

Investigations

- Metabolic acidosis with an increased anion gap *plus*
- Serum D-lactate >3 mmol/L (NB: the renal threshold for D-lactate is lower than for L-lactate)

Management

- Decrease enteral feed rates or carbohydrate intake
- Correction of acidosis
- Consider use of acetate in the PN solution
- Subsequent use of probiotics may prevent recurrence

Other complications

These include IFALD, gallstones, oxalosis, obstruction and hypertriglyceridaemia.

Important features from history

- Recurrent abdominal pain, a history of dehydration and episodes of jaundice can all reflect biliary sludge or gallstone formation
- Calcium oxalate renal stones can occur in SBS with a retained functioning colon, due to increased absorption of dietary oxalate, especially in the presence of fat malabsorption. Symptoms include acute severe abdominal pain and dysuria
- Bone health: metabolic bone disease can occur on long-term PN but fractures are uncommon. Monitor calcium and phosphate intake; vitamin D and bone density should be checked at intervals

Investigations

- Abdominal ultrasound
- Urinary oxalate and citrate
- DEXA

Management of hyperoxaluria

- Ensure adequate sodium and water intake
- Calcium supplements with meals may be helpful
- Low oxalate diet
- A low fat diet may help
- Ensure no acidosis (may require bicarbonate supplements)
- Magnesium supplements may help
- Citrate supplements if low citrate in urine
- Cholestyramine, by binding bile salts, may decrease oxalate absorption

Further reading

Bowen A, Carapetis J. Advances in the diagnosis and management of central venous access device infections in children. *Adv Exp Med Biol* 2011;697:91–106

Chalmers E, Ganesen V, Liesner R *et al.* Guideline on the investigation, management and prevention of venous thrombosis in children. *Br J Haematol* 2011;154:196–207

Cole CR, Frem JC, Schmotzer B et al. The rate of bloodstream infection is high in infants with short bowel syndrome: relationship with small bowel bacterial overgrowth, enteral feeding, and inflammatory and immune responses. *J Pediatr* 2010;156:941–947.e1

Dobson R, McGuckin C, Walker G et al. Cycled enteral antibiotics reduce sepsis rates in paediatric patients on long-term parenteral nutrition for intestinal failure. *Aliment Pharmacol Ther* 2011;34:1005–1011.

Greenberg RG, Moran C, Ulshen M, Smith PB, Benjamin DK Jr, Cohen-Wolkowiez M. Outcomes of catheter-associated infections in pediatric patients with short bowel syndrome. *J Pediatr Gastroenterol Nutr* 2010;50:460–462

Koletzko B, Goulet O, Hunt J, Krohn K, and Shamir R for the Parenteral Nutrition Guidelines Working Group. Guidelines on Paediatric Parenteral Nutrition of the European Society of Paediatric Gastroenterology, Hepatology and Nutrition (ESPGHAN) and the European Society for Clinical Nutrition and Metabolism (ESPEN), Supported by the European Society of Paediatric Research (ESPR). *J Parenter Gastroenterol Nutr* 2005;41:S1–S87

Peña de la Vega L, Lieske JC, Milliner D, Gonyea J, Kelly DG. Urinary oxalate excretion increases in home parenteral nutrition patients on a higher intravenous ascorbic acid dose *J Parenter Enteral Nutr* 2004;28:435

Quigley EM. Microflora modulation of motility. *J Neurogastroenterol Motil* 2011;17:140–147.

van Ommen CH, Tabbers MM. Catheter-related thrombosis in children with intestinal failure and long-term parenteral nutrition: how to treat and to prevent? *Thromb Res* 2010;126:465–470

Parenteral nutrition: weaning

Most children will not require life-long PN and should be weaned as bowel function returns to normal.

How to wean

- When thresholds of tolerance have not yet been reached, i.e. stools <6stools/day with no nappy rash, or stoma output <25–30mL/kg/day,then enteral feeds can be gradually increased
- Once a threshold is reached and stool/stoma output increases, maintain feeds at last tolerated amount with no further increase in feeds until improvement in output
- Strategies to aid weaning include use of loperamide and codeine phosphate, and trial of cycled enteral antibiotics or cholestyramine (if no ileo-caecal valve)
- Consider commencing weaning foods if >4 months old
- Parenteral nutrition (PN) should be cut back as tolerated. Consider cycling over fewer hours and decreased number of days per week as feeds increase

Which enteral feed?

- Hydrolysed protein is more easily absorbed than whole protein and stimulates enterocyte proliferation and hypertrophy
- A high percentage of medium-chain triglycerides (MCTs) allows for alternative fat pathways for absorption, especially if bile acid secretion is low

Practical Approach to Paediatric Gastroenterology, Hepatology and Nutrition, First Edition.
Deirdre Kelly, Ronald Bremner, Jane Hartley, and Diana Flynn.
© 2014 John Wiley & Sons, Ltd. Published 2014 by John Wiley & Sons, Ltd.

- Partially hydrólysed formulae are usually less osmolar than amino acid formulae, but if protein hydrolysates fail, a trial of an amino acid formula should be considered
- Carbohydrate content of a feed can also limit tolerance, and in this case, a modular feed with gradually increasing carbohydrate and/or fat can be trialled

Outcome

Many children with short bowel syndrome (SBS) and even enteropathy can be weaned off PN over time. Small bowel transplantation should be reserved for those with life-threatening complications as survival on home parenteral nutrition (HPN) is excellent.

Home parenteral nutrition

Home parenteral nutrition (HPN) provision aims to provide nutritional support for children with intestinal failure outside of hospital.

Indications

Permanent or long-term intestinal failure where the gut is insufficient to meet nutritional requirements and where acute medical care is no longer required and a stable PN prescription can be achieved.

Investigations

Investigations are as for intestinal failure (see Chapter 44), with intensity of monitoring depending on factors such as diarrhoea and active weaning onto enteral feeds

Before consideration for HPN several conditions must be achieved:

- It must be possible to train parents or other carers in PN administration or ensure that adequate nursing support for this is provided
- Training must also be given for management of accidental line removal and basic resuscitation
- A home visit is necessary to ensure the family home is suitable and can be adapted so that PN can be administered safely and hygienically
- Factors that need to be considered include a separate bedroom for the child; adequate number of plugs; space for storage of PN, including a fridge; mixer taps on a suitable nearby sink for handwashing and safe door handles to avoid catching lines and risking line removal

Practical Approach to Paediatric Gastroenterology, Hepatology and Nutrition, First Edition.
Deirdre Kelly, Ronald Bremner, Jane Hartley, and Diana Flynn.
© 2014 John Wiley & Sons, Ltd. Published 2014 by John Wiley & Sons, Ltd.

Management

Parents are usually trained by a specialist nutrition nurse. Training takes several weeks and length of time to achieve competence depends on many factors, including parental availability and how quickly techniques can be learned.

Outcome

The outcome for HPN is excellent, with most children who go home on PN surviving into adulthood. The risk of central line infection is decreased on leaving hospital and quality of life is acceptable, with children attending school and social activities. PN can be provided for family holidays including travel abroad. Adolescents will require tailoring of PN to support their social life, including changing start and stop times to allow them to mix with their peers in the evenings.

Enteral tube feeding

Enteral tube feeding is used to ensure safe and sufficient nutrition where oral feeding is dangerous or insufficient to meet nutritional demands (Table 49.1 and Table 49.2).

The use of enteral feeding should include a plan for weaning onto a normal diet, unless the indications for long-term feeding are clear, e.g. long-term neurodevelopmental delay with non-safe swallow. Even so, revisiting safe swallow over time may allow some oral intake (see Table 49.1).

Types of tube and usage

Nasogastric (NG)
- Should be considered initially where gastric feeds are required
- Placement:
  - Measurement of approximate length for NG tube placement is determined by measuring from the ear to the corner of the mouth + mouth to xiphoid. Appropriate placement should be determined either radiologically (between 11th and 12th thoracic vertebrate) or by checking pH. If pH is <4 this is a reliable indicator of position in the stomach
  - Difficulties arise in children requiring long-term NG tubes who are on acid suppression as recurrent use of X-rays may result in high radiation dose over time

Nasojejunal
- Useful especially in the critical care setting or for short-term use in superior mesenteric artery (SMA) syndrome

Practical Approach to Paediatric Gastroenterology, Hepatology and Nutrition, First Edition.
Deirdre Kelly, Ronald Bremner, Jane Hartley, and Diana Flynn.
© 2014 John Wiley & Sons, Ltd. Published 2014 by John Wiley & Sons, Ltd.

Table 49.1 Indications for gastric feeding

Indication	Rationale
Intestinal failure	Continuous feeds allow slow increase in feed and maximum time for enterocyte contact with nutrients
Poor oral tolerance of artificial feeds	Allows treatment to be continued effectively, e.g. modulen for Crohn's, elemental feed for food allergy
Unsafe swallow	Allows safe enteral feeding or, if swallow partially effective and food intake slow (>30 minutes/meal) allows some oral diet and the rest by tube
Other feeding difficulties, e.g. heart failure or respiratory distress in infancy	Allows ongoing enteral nutrition when oral intake likely to be poor or unsafe
Poor appetite during disease treatment, e.g. oncology patients	Allows enteral nutrition to continue

Table 49.2 Indications for jejunal feeds

Indication	Rationale
Upper gastrointestinal tract dysmotility Recurrent vomiting or delayed gastric emptying	Bypass stomach
Superior mesenteric artery syndrome	Bypasses area of narrowing in duodenum

- However, they do migrate back into the stomach and in younger children or with vomiting may become dislodged

Gastrostomy
- For longer term gastric feeding (>2 months)
- Placement:
  ○ Can be inserted endoscopically (PEG), laparoscopically or via open procedure

- PEG tubes can be placed with experience even in very small infants (down to about 3 kg
- Can be placed with minimal complications in patients with Crohn's
- Open placement of gastrostomy tubes may be necessary where there is scoliosis or other risk factors
- Contraindications for PEG: significant clotting disorders, ascites, peritonitis

Jejunostomy

Direct jejunal insertion or more often gastro-jejunal (G-J) tube with the advantage that the gastric port allows venting/aspiration of stomach contents.

Investigations

- Prior to gastrostomy insertion, assess degree (if any) of reflux with a pH study and exclude malrotation with a barium meal.
- A trial of NG feeding to assess potential benefits is usually indicated

Management (Table 49.3)

- Immediate post insertion:
  - Ensure adequate pain relief
  - Monitor for discomfort, bleeding, vomiting, fever and signs of peritonitis
  - Feeds can usually be commenced within 24 hours once bowel sounds present
  - Clean site daily
- Longer term:
  - Continue to keep site clean
  - Gastrostomies and jejunostomies require regular turning through 360 degrees to prevent buried bumper syndrome (gastrostomy becoming embedded in gastric wall)
  - The water in a balloon will need to be changed occasionally: see individual tube type
  - Gastrostomies need to be changed occasionally: see local protocol
  - Regular anthropometry to ensure appropriate calorie intake

Equipment required at home

- Handwashing facilities
- Tray
- Gloves

Table 49.3 Complications of gastrostomy/jejunostomy

Complication	Presentation	Management
Infection	Site looks red and is sticky/smelly	Topical or oral antibiotics
Overgranulation		Maxitrol or silver nitrate applied to granulation tissue only
Leakage	Gastric/jejunal contents causing excoriation of abdominal wall	Ensure correct size of tube, gastric balloon inflated correctly
Tube blockage	Usually due to inadequate flushing or very thick medication	Use only liquid medications; flush with warm water
Tube falls out		Pass either a replacement tube if possible or NG tube through the site and secure until formal replacement to prevent track closing
Constipation		High fibre feeds
Gastric upset	Nausea, vomiting, abdominal cramps, diarrhoea	Ensure feed not too cold; rate may need decreased
Gas in stomach	Abdominal distension	Gastrostomy may require venting (aspirate air from the gastrostomy)

Note: dental hygiene is important as gum disease may develop if the mouth is no longer used for eating food.

- Alco-wipes
- Chlorhexidine
- Bacteriology swabs
- Saline
- Syringes

Feeding using an enteral tube

- Choice of feed depends on the reason for insertion
- Lower concentrations of feed and the use of continuous feeds is recommended for jejunal tubes to decrease the risk of diarrhoea

Long-term enteral feeding can be extremely difficult for parents, as they are no longer providing food for their child. Parents may request blended or puréed food that they prepare themselves instead of liquid feeds. This is not standard practice and further studies are required in this area.

Most liquid medications can be given via a gastrostomy.

Information: Role of gastrostomy nurse

- To prepare the family for the procedure
- To ensure optimal aftercare of gastrostomy, to teach families how to avoid and recognise complications and to give advice in case of complications
- To train school staff to administer feeds and to be able to recognise and prevent complications
- To change tubes when required (those not needing to be changed under anaesthetic) and to teach families how to do so where appropriate

---

Key web links

Caring for children and young people in the community receiving enteral tube feeding. Best practice statement 2007 NHS Scotland. Includes summary of checking position of NG tubes and daily care of gastrostomy and jejunal tubes, and administering feeds: http://www .cen.scot.nhs.uk/files/12j-nastrogastric-and-gastronomy-tube-feeding -for-children-being-cared-for-in-the-community.pdf

ESPEN guidelines on use of PEG tubes: http://www.espen.org/ documents/PEG.pdf

Gastrostomy feeding guidelines for patients and carers: http://www .fresenius-kabi.co.uk/files/EN00322_-_Feka_PEG_aftercare _booklet_August_2012.pdf and http://www.fresenius-kabi.co.uk/ files/EN00321_Balloon_Booklet_April10.pdf

NHS Scotland guidelines for adults with gastrostomy tubes (although for adults, includes a useful algorithm for administration of medications, and table of complications at insertion and post insertion): http://www.healthcareimprovementscotland.org/previous_ resources/best_practice_statement/gastrostomy_tube_insertion.aspx

http://www.healthcareimprovementscotland.org/previous_resources/
best_practice_statement/enteral_tube_feeding.aspx

Setting up feeding pumps: http://www.youtube.com/watch?v=1KgklF
g8ekg&feature=related

PEG placement (adults): http://www.youtube.com/watch?v
=hSv4FOwZ9kQ

Nutrition in cystic fibrosis

CHAPTER 50

Specific nutritional needs

Children with cystic fibrosis (CF) have several reasons to require close nutritional management:

- Increased resting energy expenditure (REE) from chronic inflammation and recurrent chest infections
- Anorexia
- Fat malabsorption secondary to pancreatic exocrine insufficiency. This is exacerbated by CF liver disease. 90% of children with CF will have pancreatic insufficiency by age 1 year
- Vitamin deficiency is common, and vitamin supplementation is needed from birth. Parenteral preparations may be required
- Pancreatic endocrine insufficiency and the development of diabetes mellitus is common and complicates the need for high calorie intake

A nutritional scoring system is now available.

There needs to be close nutritional monitoring in infancy where growth is rapid. Optimal nutrition in early life may be associated with fewer respiratory infections: BMI at 2 years of age is correlated with pulmonary function.

Breast-feeding may also confer some protection, but may not provide sufficient calories, particularly after the first 1–2 months of age.

Investigations

- Faecal elastase: a reliable measure of pancreatic insufficiency
- Height, weight and skinfold thickness
- Vitamin A, D, E, coagulation: need regular monitoring
- Urinary sodium: sodium may be lost in sweat and if sodium stores are low growth may be poorer

Practical Approach to Paediatric Gastroenterology, Hepatology and Nutrition, First Edition.
Deirdre Kelly, Ronald Bremner, Jane Hartley, and Diana Flynn.
© 2014 John Wiley & Sons, Ltd. Published 2014 by John Wiley & Sons, Ltd.

Management

- Exocrine pancreatic enzyme replacement:
  - Adequate meal and snack-time replacement of enzymes is important for growth and good nutritional status
  - In infancy it can be given with feeds
  - Note that a maximum dose of lipase of 10 000 units/kg/day (and 2500 units/kg/meal) should not be exceeded, due to the risk of fibrosing colonopathy. This risk is higher in infancy
  - If enzyme replacements are not given, then zinc may also be malabsorbed and supplements can be given if growth remains poor despite increased calorie intake
- Behavioural issues with food aversion have been reported in children with CF, and strategies can be given to families to encourage an oral diet

Further reading

Cystic Fibrosis Foundation, Borowitz D, Robinson KA *et al*. Cystic Fibrosis Foundation evidence-based guidelines for management of infants with cystic fibrosis. *J Pediatr* 2009;155 (6 Suppl):S73–93

Debray D, Kelly D, Houwen R, Strandvik B, Colombo C. Best practice guidance for the diagnosis and management of cystic fibrosis-associated liver disease. *J Cyst Fibros* 2011;10 (Suppl 2):S29–36

Jadin SA, Wu GS, Zhang Z, *et al*. Growth and pulmonary outcomes during the first 2 y of life of breastfed and formula-fed infants diagnosed with cystic fibrosis through the Wisconsin Routine Newborn Screening Program. *Am J Clin Nutr* 2011;93:1038–1047

Sermet-Gaudelus I, Mayell SJ, Southern KW; European Cystic Finrosis Society (ECFS), Neonatal Screening Working Group. Guidelines on the early management of infants diagnosed with cystic fibrosis following newborn screening. *J Cyst Fibros* 2010;9:323–329

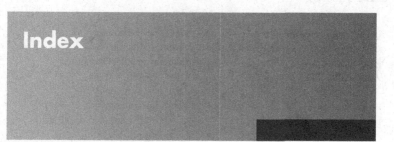

Index

Page numbers relating to Algorithms or Figures will be in *italics*, while those referring to Tables will be in **bold**

Practical Approach to Paediatric Gastroenterology, Hepatology and Nutrition, First Edition.
Deirdre Kelly, Ronald Bremner, Jane Hartley, and Diana Flynn.
© 2014 John Wiley & Sons, Ltd. Published 2014 by John Wiley & Sons, Ltd.

Printed in the United States
By Bookmasters